ENDORSEMENTS

"In his compelling book DHEAlthy: Never Get Old, the author boldly explores the possibility of slowing—or even halting—the aging process through supplementation of the hormone DHEA. Blending engaging personal anecdotes from his nearly three-decade-long self-experimentation with insightful discussions on human biology and evolution, he presents a passionate and thought-provoking argument for DHEA's rejuvenating potential.

Particularly striking is the author's enthusiasm and dedication to harnessing the body's natural mechanisms to maintain youthfulness and vitality. His clear, straightforward narrative and inspiring personal successes offer readers practical guidance and a meaningful opportunity to reflect deeply on their own health and wellness journeys.

While claims of reversing aging may initially seem ambitious, the author's meticulous documentation and thoughtful analysis provide substantial material for consideration. Readers interested in alternative health practices, evolutionary biology, or methods for enhancing vitality will find this book highly stimulating.

Ultimately, 'DHEAlthy: Never Get Old' fosters an open conversation around aging, encouraging readers—and even extending its potential to pets—to reconsider the assumed inevitability of aging. Although any health-related approach should be pursued in consultation with healthcare professionals, the author's sincerity and detailed observations make this book valuable to ongoing dialogues about longevity, health, and well-being."

~Janice Konstantinidis, author, poet, Post-Grad Diploma in Education, U. of Canberra

"If you think you know everything about keeping aging at bay, you haven't read Leonard Carpenter's DHEA book or met the man himself. I guarantee it will be a revelation."

~ Harvey Ardman, author of teleplays and novels including **Hello Earth**.

"After reading DHEAlthy and meeting Leonard, I was deeply impressed — not only by the man himself but by the powerful message of his book. I began following his regimen, and the results have been incredible. I feel better than ever. If you're searching for the secret to longevity, this is the book for you. Highly recommended!"

~ *Gary B, Patron of the Arts & Adventure Rider, DHEA user*

"Leonard Carpenter has found the Fountain of Youth – and it's legal, safe, and readily available! If you knew this groovy guy, who has more energy, strength, and stamina in his late 70's than most people I know under 30, you'd drink the Kool-Aid, too. A fascinating read!"

~ *Melanie Senn, Educator, reporter, author of **Murray, A Novel***

"Carpenter's book is an autobiographical celebration of the many benefits he's experienced since supplementing his dehydroepiandrosterone (DHEA) at age 48. His story is not unique, yet the benefits of this important human repair signal still remain a secret to many. Despite over 10,000 studies about DHEA readily available to the public, it remains an enigma to many of my medical doctor colleagues. I have been supplementing DHEA to get into the health zone for women of 250-350 µg per deciliter for women for over two decades. My husband has been supplementing to get his level into the health zone for men of 350-400 µg/dL for 38 years. My hope for Mr. Carpenter's book is that readers use his bibliography to learn more, get their

DHEA-sulfate levels tested, and supplement as appropriately to optimize the repair in their body, promoting balanced hormone levels as they age. I appreciate his mindfulness about the importance of working with one's medical team to get the best outcome. People can find a hormone balancing specialist in their community by contacting their local Compounding Pharmacy and asking for a list of providers that are well educated in this area."

~ *Natalie Kather, MD, Family and Anti-Aging Medicine; Hormone Balancing Specialist and Co-Author of* **The Metabolic Makeover: It's All About Energy!**

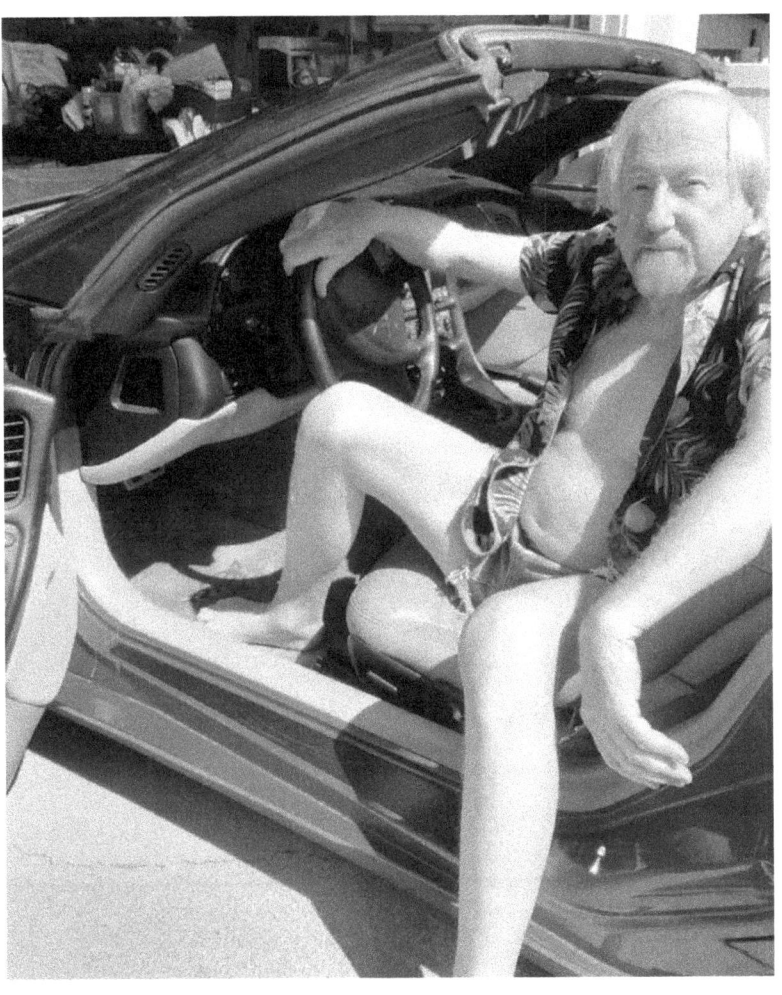

DHEAlthy: Never Get Old

How I Live Infinitely Without

Aging

by Leonard Carpenter

Preface by Dr. Doug Garland

Neither the publisher nor the author is engaged in rendering professional advice or services to the individual reader. The ideas, procedures, and suggestions contained in this book are not intended as a substitute for consulting with your physician. All matters regarding your health require medical supervision. Neither the author nor the publisher shall be liable or responsible for any loss or damage allegedly arising from any information or suggestion in this book.

*The information contained herein is **not** presented with the intention of diagnosing or prescribing, but is offered only as information for use in maintaining and promoting health in cooperation with a physician. In the event that the information presented in this book is used without a physician's approval, the individual will be diagnosing for himself. No responsibility is assumed by the author, publisher, or distributors of this publication for use of the information contained herein in lieu of a doctor's services. No guarantees of any kind are made for the performance or effectiveness of the preparations mentioned in this publication.*

More information at www.dhealthy.net

ISBNs:
eBook - 979-8-9898007-6-6
Paperback - 979-8-9898007-7-3
Hardback - 979-8-9898007-9-7
Audio - 979-8-9898007-8-0

Published by Siafu Productions 2025
www.siafuproductions.com

TABLE OF CONTENTS

Preface by Dr. Doug Garland

PREFACE BY DR. DOUGLAS GARLAND, M.D.

This book contains an inexpensive do-it-yourself formula for life extension, pioneered by a unique, independent experimenter, Leonard Carpenter, also known on TikTok as Leo the Immortal. The regimen is based on Leonard's revolutionary theory of aging. After following his unique daily routine between 1996 and 2025, he claims it has preserved his health, youth and stamina from his prime of life at age 48 and can possibly maintain it forever, far past his current age of 77.

Having met Leo only recently, I've never taken part in his experiment. But as a medical professional, I see no reason why it can't work. He's sold me on it, though I may be too old to benefit.

Leo, not being a physician or a health professional, cannot give medical advice or prescribe treatment for any disease or injury. He can only describe his own experiences and results, and let readers judge the validity of his theory. My position is much the same.

However, anyone trying this supplement long-term should consult their physician and continue with regular medical treatments and checkups. It is not a substitute for prescriptions, although it could, over time, relieve the need for later treatment.

I, as an MD and orthopedic surgeon, have commented on the quality and credibility of Leo's claims. I can provide relevant insights, without necessarily recommending his or any other procedure.

Leonard's simple routine is based on a daily pill to supplement a single hormone substance, dehydroepiandrosterone (DHEA), just enough to maintain its youthful adult blood level. He concludes that every human body's scheduled, natural depletion of DHEA is the sole cause of all the ancient ills and complaints of aging, a loss leading

inexorably to death.

Leo's breakthrough is that—rather than death being an

inevitable result of wear and tear, tissue failure, and immune

failure against specific diseases—aging and death are a

biologically programmed self-destruct attained in the process

of evolution. He now reveals that all humans, physicians, and

the medical industry have subscribed to a false paradigm, the

age-old assumption that our death is due to the inevitable

breakdown of our bodies. Instead, he demonstrates, death is

due to another cause.

If true, this is a radical insight that will revolutionize

anti-aging and mortality. There may be controversy, since so

far, Leo is a lone experimenter, the sole poster-boy for

immortality. It may take five years to test his hypothesis on

rats, and decades longer to fully validate it in human studies.

But for now, since DHEA is non-prescription, uncontrolled in the US, and natural to the human body with almost no undesired side effects, others may soon try out his routine to gain its immediate benefits of improved mood, health and vigor, plus the longevity that Leo calls "Living Indefinitely."

I met Leo in 2023 at a writing workshop while promoting my own literary work, most recently The Tall Poppy Syndrome, a study of human behavior which analyzes and accounts for many of the peaks and reversals that shape our history, culture and social media. After 37 years as an orthopedic surgeon in California, I encountered the Tall Poppy phenomenon in Australia and decided to pursue and popularize it here, resulting in an easy read available on Amazon.

Also, from my career dealing with bones, joints, muscles, tendons, blood circulation and nerves in the context of injury, disease and universal human aging, I'm uniquely qualified to recognize the deeper design and function of the human organism as revealed here in Leonard Carpenter's work.

Leo, not being a physician or health professional, cannot give medical advice or prescribe treatment for any disease or injury. I agreed to support Leo with his book by helping him with scientific methodology and providing expertise regarding medical information. I can't make any recommendations related to DHEA supplementation.

Dr. Douglas Garland, MD

San Luis Obispo, California

July 1, 2024

CHAPTER 1

THE BREAKTHROUGH

I am here to announce a revolution in human existence and medical science. This book proclaims my discovery of cheap, easy immortality for those not already impaired by serious disease, damage, or decline from aging. I have continued my dosage daily for the last 28 of my 76 years and now can proclaim, I'm not physically aging, and can potentially extend my life and health forever. "To Eternity, and Beyond!"

This secret of mine has been disclosed to very few. And most of those, quite predictably, haven't believed me or practiced it. I've finally reached an age where my continued youthfulness should be evident even to skeptics. But now I'm in the sad position of seeing my oldest, dearest friends suffering and failing from age, facing inexorable death. Yet I must move forward with new generations to an enlightened future, where humans can live and thrive without decline, like immortal gods.

It all began when, quite logically inspired by a radio medical interview in 1996, at age 48, I began a single daily pill dosage that offsets the gradual decline of aging. This is based on a fundamental biological principle, first discovered by me, which can benefit humans and our pets.

Having followed my own unique dosage for 28 years, I now at age 76 have the same mood, energy and strength levels I had in my prime at age 48. My dog Lizzie at 11, (77 dog years) on a proportional dose, is still frisky and puppyish. Strange to think that my Husky/McNab mix is statistically older than I am, but equally young!

The pill we take is cheap, safe and non-prescription. It's just a supplement of a simple molecule, a pre-hormone that plays a vital role in our youthful, healthy bodies.

Due mostly to shallow, ancient assumptions about aging and death still retained by most everyone else, I am, to my knowledge, the first and only person to "think outside the box" and proclaim this scientific miracle. Therefore, I claim the sole credit and recognition for my epochal discovery.

This book sets forth the basic information I've learned or formulated in my own experimentation. However, I'm not a medical professional and I cannot recommend any dosage or treatment for anyone else. Please consult your doctor, as I've always done, and read this book to understand the revolution in medical care that I believe is soon to occur based on my findings.

Once proven, this brilliant "paradigm shift" can transform human life and thought, make most of us immortal, and open the way to a splendid future – IF, and only if, we can overcome the looming threats to our earthly life and biosphere.

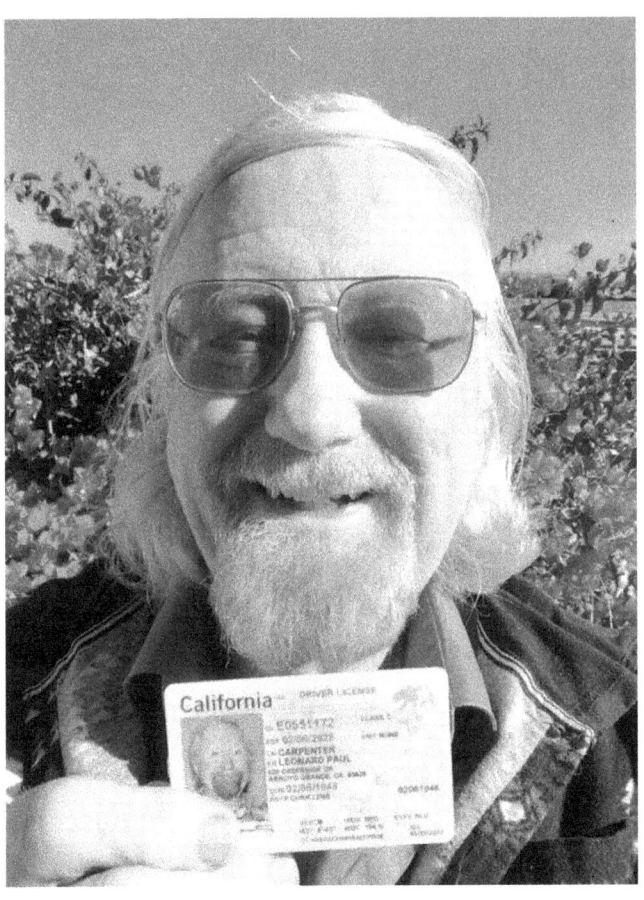

CHAPTER 2

PRECURSOR

(*asterisks refer to research pages, listed by Chapter at the end

of the bibliography)

DHEA stands for dehydro-epiandrosterone—a big word,

the antidisestablishmentarianism of drug names! Here, for

short, I'll refer to DHEA as "D." My web address for it is

dhealthy.net. Neat, yes?

(Note: DHEA should not be confused with DHA, a fish oil

extract; nor here, with Vitamin D.)

DHEA naturally occurs in abundance in young mammal

bodies. So, no allergy or overdose involving D is likely. It later

declines with age, * but by what causative process, no one yet

knows. The regulator that chokes off D likely exists

somewhere deep in the animal brain or pre-brain.

Our D is a simple molecule produced mainly in the adrenals—that is, in the adrenal cortex of the two adrenal glands located on top of the human kidneys. After maturity, their D production declines.

This decline seems strange, since the adrenals don't appear to atrophy with age. General adrenal insufficiency, called Addison's Disease, is a rare condition that can emerge at any age. The loss of D with aging has perhaps wrongly been called "adrenopause*," comparable to the loss of ovulation in female menopause. (Yet the adrenals don't pause or fail to produce cortisol and adrenaline hormones at later ages. So, they are not, in a broad sense, failing.)

Some D in lesser amounts is also produced locally in the male testes, female ovaries, skin, and brain. It's unclear to me if the production from these sources is also lost or reduced with aging. But production in other tissues is probably local, and far from adequate to offset the loss of adrenal D.

In the bloodstream, DHEA mainly takes the form of DHEAS, a sulfate which has a longer half-life and can be converted back to DHEA in the tissues*. So, in routine blood tests, it's more meaningful to test for DHEAS levels than for DHEA.

D's main function is as is the "precursor," the essential ingredient, of all the sex hormones including testosterone, estrogen, progesterone, androgen and others. D is a "mother hormone" available in the blood to be converted to these other substances on demand, as needed by various tissues of the body.

DHEA—as a hormone or not—also vitally aids and regulates immune protection and tissue repair. It stabilizes mood and has other vital functions. * And now, most critically, we see that D's programmed decline heralds all the ills of aging.

D is very similar to the cholesterol molecule, but it doesn't clog the arteries. In fact, it may reduce the chance of clogged arteries and associated heart problems. Some studies suggest that LOW DHEA levels are linked to fatal heart attacks in men and may be a risk factor for coronary heart disease and stroke*. Other studies have shown that increased D levels may reduce atherosclerosis and blockage of the heart's arteries.

In my theory, as borne out by personal experience, DHEA supplementation can stop the body's slow breakdown leading to inevitable death. By orally replacing my lost D, I've been able to maintain youthful health results. By medical treatment and other supplements, I'm even able to repair older damage suffered before taking DHEA, with the D likely aiding in this, too.

Hormones are usually released into the bloodstream in early morning. D seems to sustain a healthy level throughout the day, so whatever my D dose, I take it with all my pills in the morning.

In adult human blood, D reaches its peak concentration at about age 20. Then it declines gradually with age. As it fades, its ABSENCE becomes a dire "precursor" to disease, injury and death, most all the ills to which the mortal flesh is heir. This genetic trait appears to exist in all animals that have a natural lifespan. Like sex, it was evolved early-on to accelerate evolution, which is the adaptation of animal species to changing conditions (see Chapter 8.)

CHAPTER 3

SAFE AND LEGAL

There is a vast amount of research on DHEA reported in scientific papers. The results have been summarized in expert books, so I provide a bibliography. I haven't followed all the studies closely. But to my knowledge, there haven't been dangers or severe side effects of D reported*. One exception: the only significant risk of DHEA might be, if the patient already has an active cancer. Since D promotes hormone activity, it could conceivably speed cancer's growth. (Of course, D is already in our bodies, less so as we age; and youth are LESS prone to cancer.) But cancer patients should not supplement DHEA without first consulting their oncologist.

Another caution is that DHEA should NOT be taken by women who are pregnant or lactating or by children. D is present in infants, but excess amounts might affect the growth and development of the child.

The main cautions I've seen quoted are cosmetic ones – mainly, the possibility of unwanted hair growth in women, or accelerated hair loss. I experienced a pimple after taking my first D dose for a few days, so I immediately cut my daily dose in half, with no recurrence but with continued benefits of mood and energy. It would seem that any unwanted reactions can be corrected by reducing the dose or discontinuing… if one prefers instead to face the inevitable pangs of aging and death.

This is unlike the known risks and side-effects of specific hormone supplements, such as anabolic steroids. Alone, by supplementing only D, the raw material "progenitor" of all the sex-differentiated hormones, I've trusted my body to maintain and generate the same hormonal balance that made up my adult physiology, physique, and personality. If you ask anyone about me, they'll say my basic character, moods and temperament have not changed noticeably. Nor has my appearance, except I'm a bit leaner. I believe D is safe and I haven't noticed any ill effects except oily skin or pimples, soon corrected.

To the best of my knowledge, DHEA is restricted in the United Kingdom countries, including Canada and Australia. It may be available there under prescription, and I don't know if legal constraints are enforced. In Europe, D is known as Prasterone and is used for female hormone replacement after menopause, often as a vaginal suppository or cream.

In some US sports, D may be regarded as a banned steroid. However, in past decades, I've heard it used as a legal defense against unproven charges of injectable steroid abuse. I've met athletes who take it orally to improve general health and stamina. And DHEA is a minor ingredient in many common "wellness" pills, though likely not in large enough quantities to provide the revolutionary benefits that I proclaim.

For years, I purchased D pills as a pharmaceutical supplement in chain drugstores or vitamin stores. It has been broadly available since the 1990's as a white powder in tablets or capsules, usually in 25 mg. size, with fillers to make the pills bigger and easier to handle or swallow.

For years, I bought the Schiff brand, then store brands, usually for about $20 for 60 pills, which at the start would last me 120 days. The advantage of tablets over capsules is that I can cut them in half for a fairly precise, comfortable dosage. And those first Schiff tabs were scored with a line down the middle for splitting. The mixing of DHEA with rice flour or other white fillers needs to be uniform and constant in pharmaceutical equipment to equalize the dosage in pills and half-pills.

How do I know that it was? Because of my body's remarkable sensitivity to the proper dosage. I'd notice.

But why is dosing such an issue, you ask? It's because of my unique discovery: Because of the steadily progressing decline of natural DHEA, to be effective against aging, my dosage of D had to INCREASE steadily, from month to month and year to year, to keep me youthful. If I missed a dose or if it had become insufficient, I would know it by mid-afternoon. I could feel it.

D decline accelerates; so, my incremental increase gradually grew, from 6 to 50 mg. at a time, over twenty years, step by step, as my natural D supply dropped off more steeply to zero—until in my early seventies I finally reached my current stable, satisfactory daily "plateau" dose of 600 mg. per day.

So, as my body's natural production declined, my need for supplementation grew. I progressed to buying D online from various companies in more economical 50 and 100 milligram capsules. Since age 73, my constant, "maxed-out" morning dose of 600 mg. is adequate, and I've never craved more or lacked that youthful "normal" feeling and outlook during the day.

I can pack my own capsules for convenience. Using a small pill-packing kit, a size "0" pill can hold about 200 milligrams of pure DHEA powder. So, taking three of those each morning averages out my daily dose to at least 600 to 650 milligrams, per the reading on a pocket-sized gram scale. At this level of use, the amount doesn't have to be precise each day, just sufficient.

I've recently switched to using a small scoop to obtain 600 milligrams of the pure powder that I buy, then mixing it with

water or fruit juice. It can be part of the "morning smoothie"
that many health enthusiasts like to blend. (I've never tried
taking D with coffee, since that morning caffeine boost could
have negated or replaced the sense of wellness I look for to
determine my dosage level.)

Thanks to high pharmaceutical standards, I've never bought
DHEA that proved fake or ineffective. I would have noticed a
deficiency in my mood and well-being from a substitute—as I
invariably do by mid-afternoon, if I miss my morning dose, or
if it proved insufficient due to age decline. But when buying,
one should always pay attention to the label and source to feel
sure that the contents are genuine and not overly adulterated.
To the best of my knowledge, fake or weak pills would not
provide any "placebo effect."

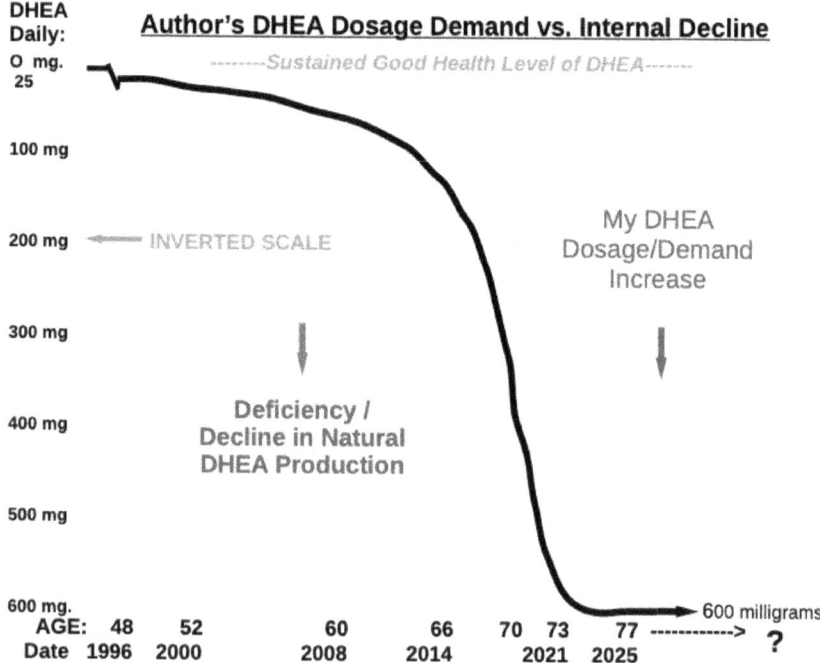

Author's DHEA Dosage Demand vs. Internal Decline

Theoretical Graph of Male & Female DHEA Production & Depletion by Dr. Shealy (see Bibliography)

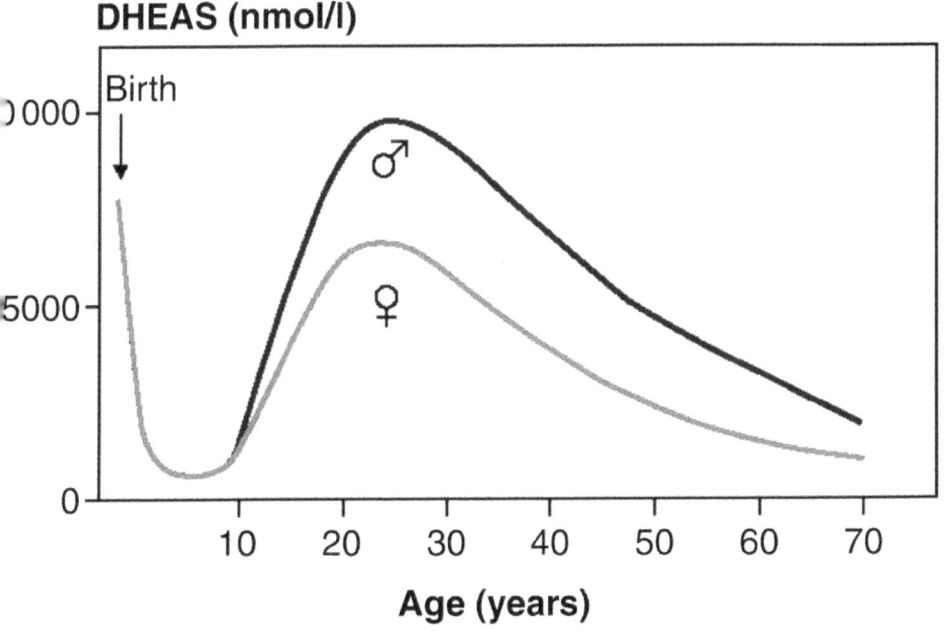

CHAPTER 4

SELF-DOSING

The above doesn't end the delicate question of dosage.

Since I'm alone in my experiment to use DHEA for longevity,

I can't be sure others would have exactly the same experience.

But I now know it works for me. I first proclaimed my method

in a 2020 Medium blog titled "Immortality Is Here," at:

https://medium.com/living-indefinitely/immortality-is-here-
4f43df1444a1

I may be lucky or gifted, but one thing may also have

helped: I didn't partake of daily stimulants. No coffee or

tobacco, and no weed or other habits to dull or intensify my

feelings and thoughts. As of 1996 I seldom drank, just

occasional beer or wine, and I'd never smoked anything except a few puffs of marijuana (which, on two occasions, were

followed by bronchitis.) I avoid even cola drinks because the

caffeine disrupts my sleep, hours later. I've lately begun using

coffee only at my bi-weekly morning writers' group, or when

traveling, jet-lagged. If I had used any daily stimulant earlier, I

might have sought after another smoke or another cup of "Joe"

for a rush, instead of pursuing my anti-aging experiment. Now

that I know its daily routine works, I can experiment cautiously

with legal stimulants, but I would not let one wean me off my

regular DHEA.

One influence I did have was my elderly mother who, over

the phone in her seventies, complained of her loss of mental

energy with aging. I used to joke with her that it was the

gasoline "energy crisis" of the Carter Presidency, 1977 to 81.

All I could do then was try and cheer her up. It wasn't enough.

When asked "How are you?" one of her favorite replies was, "Oh, if I had a gun, I'd shoot myself."

Apart from that mood complaint, Mom was an intelligent, pleasant lady. She couldn't provide a reason for her depression and was asking for help. It wasn't physical—if we went for a walk on her visits, she'd wear me out trekking the San Francisco hills. She still managed to be a positive and even enthusiastic person, sharing insights and news features. But for her, life was a quiet, patient struggle.

The insight came to me at 48, after her passing. Then I was commuting long hours weekly to LA, working late to make up for travel time and rushing home weekends to do housework for my teacher-wife. I began to recognize the feeling from what she'd described: some lack or deficiency of aging that didn't allow me the same energy and zest in overcoming daily challenges. Like my mom's malaise, it was a mystery;

probably, as we used to say, just hormonal. But I began to feel old.

Then in my LA motel, I happened to hear a radio interview with the late Dr. William Regelson, co-author of a new bestseller, The Superhormone Promise. He identified the likely cause of age-lag, a natural decline in hormones, and specifically of the "mother hormone" DHEA. So, I walked across the street to Long's Drugs and bought a bottle.

That next morning, with my first pill, I experienced a freshness, a surge of energy and well-being! No more lag and drag of advancing age. I felt normal again.

But then after a couple of days, back home in central California, my morning sensation was slightly giddy, too light-headed, feeling by afternoon like I was "wired to the ceiling." And a small pimple appeared on my cheek—good evidence that the pills were working, with stepped-up hormone activity and increasingly oily skin. But I didn't want to be that young! I adjusted my dose, immediately cutting my 25 mg. daily pills in half. Swiftly my giddiness and zit went away, but the youthful boost remained.

I stayed on that dose, about 12.5 mg. daily, for at least a year, still feeling my youthful "normal" energy level. Then, inevitably, the old listless feelings returned. Time to restore my initial dose?

But when I went back to the full 25 mg. pills, oops, I felt skittish again!

So, I began cutting my half-pills in half. I combined a half and a quarter, raising my daily intake to about 18.75 mg., or three-fourths of a full 25 mg. pill, per day. Voila, young again! It's amazing how sensitive my middle-aged body was to minute variations in hormone availability.

Then later, after a few more months, the age-lag came back. I resumed a full 25 mg. pill to feel "normal" for several more months, possibly a year or more.

Alas, I didn't record the exact dates and amounts of my dosage changes. I assumed these response times would vary considerably between different people. And, in those early years, I was far from certain my remedy would continue to work as unfailingly as it has. No friend or doctor believed or tried it, not even my wife, nor did she consult her doctor on it. She had other issues and treatments such as thyroid insufficiency, weight control, sleep apnea, gastric reflux, and coffee addiction. She was very solicitous and protective of her diseases, refusing advice from me or her doctors.

Please Note: DHEA wasn't a case of my habituation or addiction to a "drug." There was no "high;" I was just restoring a pleasant natural feeling. The added sensation of a higher or more frequent dose wasn't cumulative nor appealing, it was uncomfortable. I was increasing my optimal D dose just enough to compensate for my internal supply that was normally (but mysteriously) declining.

This practice kept me vital during the ensuing years. The tiny amounts of D involved, smaller than a pea and including a lot of filler, proved effective in stabilizing and sustaining my mood. (Although no longer fearing the specter of inevitable sickness and death may have helped.)

But all of this shows the extremely sensitive balance of a healthy, natural, middle-aged body—luckily in my case, not needing any daily meds at first or suffering any injury. Yet, even if I had been crippled or chronically ill, requiring continual medication, I believe that DHEA supplementation might have substantially mitigated or even alleviated those conditions. (But not a damaged thyroid from childbearing, like my poor wife; thyroid is a separate hormone that many elders

need to supplement separately, including me.)

And too, by my late forties, I had overcome, through

counseling and intensive self-therapy, most of my childhood

traumas and mid-life angst, since the death of my beloved

Mom, and the estrangement and loss of dear old Dad (who,

after nurturing me, sought to break up my happy marriage.) So,

my only emotional issues were the usual, intermittent

challenges of career, kids, family health, finances and

creativity (i.e., rejection slips) all of which I could handle

smoothly on DHEA, without undue brooding.

That pattern, of rigorously maintaining my D dosage and,

when it felt inadequate, increasing it by ever-greater

increments of 12 to 25 or 50 milligrams, continued for me over

the next twenty years. My last increase, in about 2019, was by

50 mg., going from 550 to 600 mg. per day. Since then, I've

felt no shortage, which leads me to believe that I'm now replacing all my youthful D production, that has declined to near zero. Without supplementation, that decline could be catastrophic in its effect on my mood, immune resistance, tissue repair, energy, metabolism, bone strength and size, digestion, and other vital processes mediated by hormones. Take every senior's advice and never get old!

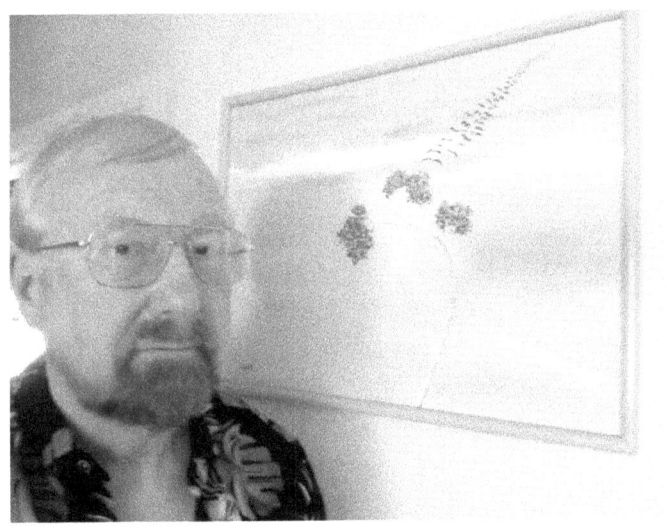

Leo's Retirement painting by Len Wise

CHAPTER 5

WHAT IS AGING?

To my way of thinking, the aging process is a biologically scheduled breakdown of tissues, defenses, and metabolism. It has evolved in humans to guarantee death within a fifty-year period between, say, ages 50 and 100, with few and very limited exceptions in human history.

Yet according to universal assumptions, advanced aging is the result of inexorable breakdowns, accrued damage and system failures, all unavoidable with age—but which many of us seek to prevent or delay by healthy habits, treatments, supplements and exercises.

Most everyone has a pet theory or habit that she or he feels can defer aging and death, be it some favorite food or drink, a diet plan, a stimulant or intoxicant, essential oils, or just a mental outlook that remains stubbornly youthful. Others rely on religion, reincarnation, yoga, spiritualism or meditation to extend life or restore it after death. But no method so far has prolonged provable life after about 125 years, with starkly evident aging decline taking place 50 to 75 years before that.

My own observation and objection to this is, that human and animal bodies are marvels of precision (except in the case of genetic flaws or dysfunctions, that mostly are evident from birth, if not fatal). A genetically healthy, well-nourished human specimen can maintain or even increase its strength, agility, fertility, intellect, and well-being into the forties and beyond.

During the first half of life, disease resistance, healing, recovery from hardship and trauma are all possible. The body maintains itself by correcting injury, illness, mild poisoning, and most notably, cancer, with built-in safeguards. Cancers, as the most frequent and destructive form of malfunction, are blocked or corrected many times daily by an active immune system. Nowadays, operable or fatal cancers are generally seen as the result of unusual stress, prolonged toxic exposure, solar or more severe radiation exposure, or some other extreme factor, including the chemical and mechanical innovations of modern life.

What I mean to say is, the body can splendidly function and protect itself for decades, up to its best "prime" years of life. Why does it then, past that age, begin to fail painfully and universally—a change which just happens to coincide with the end of fertility and childbearing in the female? Can this too be anything, but a timed, pre-programmed failure built into our wondrous natural organism?

The Bible allots us three-score and ten, that is, seventy years of life before collapse, death and transfiguration. With modern medicine and womb-to-tomb stability, we've extended that expectation to eighty-something. And before that, primitive lifespans were often short and brutal. But why NEVER anything significantly longer? Statistically based on luck and birth, the age variances should've been much larger. Random outcomes tend to include wide variants, not just one Methuselah. Aging and death were indeed inevitable, but not as a result of external/random conditions.

Yet we can't contemplate the process logically, even when death is near. How many of us, possibly a majority, deny the aging process until it hits home? The gradual, multifarious progress of aging leads us on. Everything seems to be going fine until a sudden setback, a disease or "accidental" fall occurs and suddenly it's a "cascading failure event," as they say in air crashes, with other systems crashing. By then, we're too stricken to even try and understand.

And so, why should anyone believe in my own unique denial of death? Friends dismiss my insights as impossible, eccentric—thus proving the universality of both denial and skepticism.

But it's time to face my truth. Death isn't due to "product-failure" of our flawless young bodies.

A recent bestseller by Australian researcher David Sinclair, PhD, is titled Lifespan: Why We Age – and Why We Don't Have To. It provides a number of explanations for aging, principally genetic damage due to wear and tear on telomeres, the end caps of cell DNA strands, causing the DNA to "unravel" and fail to replicate properly during cell division. Fraying, like when your shoelace tips go. This is a plausible-sounding concern about aging. And years ago, telomere loss was a concern of mine, worrying that DNA information errors would break down my tissues, prevent replication and limit my DHEA-enhanced longevity.

However, this prospect stopped being a concern when I learned that telomeres do not run out but can be routinely regenerated by a substance, telomerase, that is available in folate and other sources. For some years I supplemented folic acid, the folate sometimes given to pregnant mothers.

One substance recommended in the book to retard aging is Metformin, a diabetes drug, but the argument is based largely on anecdotal evidence from the author's father.

Other remedies discussed in Sinclair's book involve "fooling" the body into thinking that it is starving, based on the phenomenon that starvation in animals tends to slow aging and extend life. This appears to me to be a limited source of life extension at best.

In regard to my hormonal findings, I note that the word "hormone" is not indexed and apparently is never mentioned in Sinclair's book. It seems that, in Australia as a United Kingdom member, DHEA is restricted and not available for sale, import or study without special permits. This would tend to prevent any study of my theory and my findings, that:

Aging is a self-destruct, an adaptive device to speed evolution, by making room for a new random cast of the genetic dice, under new environmental conditions, to adapt and evolve. And DHEA hormone deprivation is nature's infallible kill-switch.

Until now.

CHAPTER 6

HORMONE REPLACEMENT

What I am achieving, by supplementing DHEA as its daily supply declines, is essentially, full hormone replacement.

How can one pill do this? Well, D is the key ingredient of all the sex hormones. Experience leads me to assume that:

(a) any other necessary hormones don't deplete with age, or

(b) if they do, it's because inadequate DHEA is not signaling their production.

Accordingly, by maintaining sufficient DHEA, I'm keeping all my other hormones in balance.

(The one exception I know of, as mentioned above, is Thyroid Hormone from the thyroid gland. It too does fall short in age, but can easily be replaced by a small, cheap daily pill dose. My GP physician, from his medical training, wrote me a prescription for Synthroid when I turned 70, based on age and possibly with reference to my annual blood tests.)

Another possible hormone that might naturally deplete is insulin, made by the pancreas. But although Type II adult-onset diabetes is epidemic in the US, this seems to result from eating and drinking habits rather than aging and is informally called "diabesity." I recently met a man who has a rare condition of insulin production varying drastically and unpredictably between high and low, but this came on at age 27 and clearly doesn't relate to old age or diet. For myself, I have to hope that insulin production can remain stable with a moderate diet and steady DHEA level. (If not, insulin is now easily balanced by pump or injection.)

HRT

Hormone Replacement Therapy is a common treatment, mainly for women suffering ill effects from menopause, replacing estrogen and progesterone. "ERT" normally replaces estrogen only, without progesterone, to relieve symptoms and restore hormone stability, temporarily or long-term. Both are avoided by some women out of fear that adding estrogen might increase the threat of breast cancer. But this appears to be a mistaken belief based on a misquoted Women's Health study in 2002. Any measurably increased cancer risk may be avoided by replacing estrogen but NOT progesterone. *

In my humble (male) opinion, since the Sixties when estrogen birth control pills were first used by countless women, I never heard of a cancer risk. On the contrary they're said to reduce cancer incidence and fatality. A recent book in the Bibliography addresses these concerns.

DHEA has long been used in Europe as Prasterone, mentioned above, for menopausal hormone replacement. I've also heard of DHEA being prescribed in the USA for female hormone replacement, with beneficial effects from continued use lasting long after menopause.

For women facing menopause, DHEA may warrant special dosing by a physician, or at least careful consultation. But as with any D use, adjustments are easily made by changing or deferring the dosage.

Medically, for "total" male or female hormone replacement, I gather the concerns* would be many:

(a) First, a deficiency of a certain hormone would have to be found by blood testing.

(b) Then, a suitable or bio-identical supplement would be prescribed, which might or might not be covered by health insurance.

(c) Then the desired level of hormone in the blood would have to be tested, with possible repeat tests needed.

(d) In the case of gradually declining hormones, tests would be repeated over years.

(e) The daily dosing may be interrupted for weeks, to return the blood level to "normal."

(f) New prescriptions for different doses would then be needed.

(g) Optimal dosage of some hormones may vary with changes in body weight.

(h) Some hormones such as testosterone may have to be administered by injection.

On the whole, "total" hormone replacement for essential hormones that deplete with aging would seem to be a costly, cumbersome and painful task under the care of one or more physicians.

As a brief palliative alternative, some clinics (mainly south of the border) offer health-tourists daily transfusions of blood harvested from 20-year-olds, to bestow on patients, a day at a time, the enhanced energy and sensations of extreme youth. This "blood-doping" approach is obviously costly, and perhaps risky in a health or ethical respect.

By contrast, my graduated dosages of DHEA allow the body to synthesize whatever hormones it optimally requires, keeping them in internal, individual balance with other hormones and processes. If I increase a certain hormone demand, say, by exercising heavily, I have no doubt that my body will step up production accordingly from the available supply. There's no reason to believe that my usual control and metabolic systems have been harmed by aging, as long as there's no infection or injury present.

Now, thanks to me, total hormone replacement can be cheap and easy on a do-it-yourself basis.

CHAPTER 7

IMMORTALITY

My offer to humanity of the boon of immortality is a momentous event, and one with many aspects. I feel that I must publicize it, because my wholly original insight is sure to be found or adopted by someone else. I've already put my secret out there, mainly to TikTok users who may be too young to need it. Now it goes out to eBook and print readers and audio book listeners.

I always felt it was just a matter of time before modern medicine would hit on the secret of immortality. But so far, mine is the only one that makes the necessary, logical paradigm change. And I seem to be the only one who has tested and demonstrated its worth for decades. Even my dog

Lizzie has only tried it for a couple of years, since she seemed to be slowing down. Now she's a wonder-dog.

So, there's no turning back. This great innovation will take hold of society for better or worse.

Perhaps the greatest benefit: It should remove the fear of inevitable death that drives the human intellect to desperate denial, or to remedies from ancient myth and children's stories.

But, since our religious thinking has tied morality to reward or punishment in an afterlife, release from that inevitability may cause sinners to disregard those consequences. We may have to ensure better rewards and penalties in this life to curtail sin and promote virtue. (Of course, nothing in this scientific approach denies the moral and spiritual precepts of any religion.)

My hope has been that freedom from imminent death will make humans more mindful of Earth's future and make us go easier on God's splendid treasury of biological wonders and resources. Now we may choose to continue here, instead of leaving behind a farrago of problems for our children to solve.

There may be impacts on the economy, if people live on and keep working, not opening up jobs for the next generation. (Jobs which may soon be automated anyway.) Some people will be unable to retire, if their nest eggs won't last more than a decade or two. There could be increased strain on pensions and Social Security (whose funds are robbed anyway.) Medical and insurance costs should be greatly reduced (along with the related loss and suffering) if our bodies remain healthy and youthful.

With the polycrises of climate, overpopulation, war, nuclear peril, dictators and economic collapse that loom before us, many would now say they don't want to extend their lives to face the perilous mid-century. But it's the young who are inclined and entitled to hope and work for an enjoyable, survivable future.

Of course, with the sudden drop in death rates from aging that I anticipate, the world's population may seem to explode. But this has been the steady and accelerating trend for so long that, if anything, personal immortality may be the one thing that can wake us up to reverse this primal, ignorant impulse to keep doubling and redoubling the human burden on our finite, already over-stressed planet.

So, the die is cast. If my discovery and this book are believed and accepted, a gradual but swelling change will transform life for humanity, our planet, and its species, hopefully for the better.

CHAPTER 8

EVOLUTION

Whether or not we understand or even believe in evolution, nearly all of us respect and use medical science's remedies and insights. Most antidotes were found by trial and error. My discovery was from theory, trial, and no errors as yet seen, leading to my revolutionary/evolutionary theory. But any technological medical advance, like my DHEA discovery, should satisfy scientific and evolutionary analysis.

So, my purpose in this chapter is to explain D's function from a standpoint of evolutionary science, and to surmise how it became the key to life and death. This insight should make my theory more credible and acceptable to scientific thinkers. If there seems to be any logical omission or lapse, I'd be eager to address it.

First: Why should a single molecule, DHEA, be a key to the survival or death of most animals?

That's because evolution requires a self-destruct mechanism to limit each lifespan. This effect should be obvious from human history, and from observing all animal life on Earth. But again, why?

Organisms evolve in an ecological space or "niche" that, by definition, is limited in size. To feed and reproduce, they require great structural intricacy and precision. And to thrive, they must adapt to new conditions, including environmental change and evolutionary changes in their prey and predators. They adapt best by producing new, near-identical versions of themselves: normally, new generations with gene sets re-shuffled by sexual reproduction. In case you forgot, that's the purpose of sex.

Yet obviously, the newly adapted specimens can't thrive their best while competing with old, less adaptive versions. Extreme longevity retards evolution by needless competition. Remember, nature is concerned with survival of the SPECIES, not of the individual SPECIMENS, i.e., you and me.

So, death becomes a necessity for the species to optimally survive, replicate, and evolve.

The invention of "natural death," for individuals—after a reasonable lifespan of growth, breeding, and nurture of offspring—proved to be a beneficial, even VITAL adaptation for ALL animal species.

Death is vital. It clears away old specimens so that the new, more adapted versions can thrive and reproduce. It had to be guaranteed, lest the niche soon swarm with old versions seeking to replicate. But how is this achieved? Such an invention must've been arrived at early in evolution, in the "reptile brain" or before, fundamental enough of a "find," and permanent enough to now limit the varying lifespans of all surviving animal species.

Once evolved, the self-destruct could be simple, not requiring a backup mechanism. Yet it must be deep and basic to the organism, so that it can't fail or be disabled by injury, etc., creating accidental or genetic immortals to compete with.

And too, a "sudden death" destruct, like self-poisoning, might misfire and make a species vulnerable. Such a toxin would certainly be easy for medical science to identify and treat.

So, how about hormones, the signaling compounds that trigger and regulate biological processes in animals? How better to degrade and terminate lives than by gradually choking off their hormone supply?

Best candidate: DHEA is a hormone precursor, a "mother hormone" of estrogen, testosterone and others. D also performs or triggers vital functions related to immunity, tissue repair, etc. Therefore, its depletion can be the sole, simple but reliable cause of an eventual, yet entirely certain, death.

That is how D deprivation came to be the Kill Switch, one that doesn't require a backup or fail-safe. Good news, for those of us who feel that natural human evolution is obsolete anyway.

Note: why do I say natural selection is obsolete? A friend pointed out one main cause: Medicine.

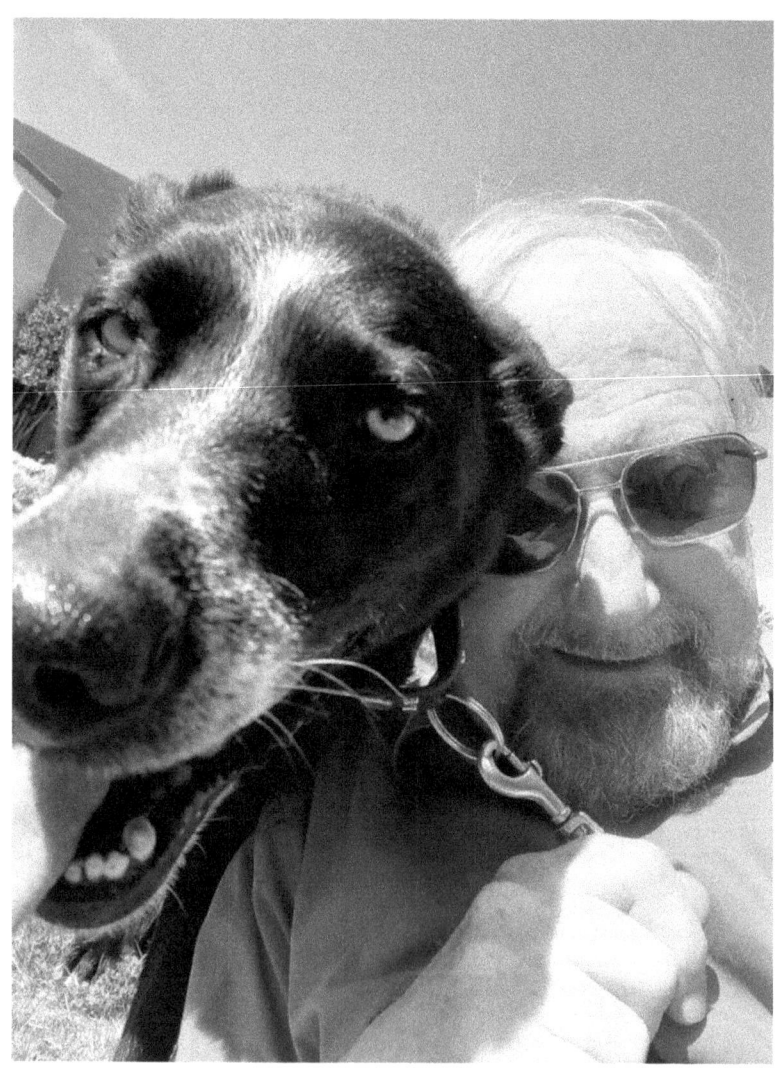

CHAPTER 9

MEDICINE

First, as stated above, I have no real medical training, except work as an orderly on a geriatric ward. I cannot reliably give medical advice or prescribe any drug or treatment for a disease. All I can do is report my own experience, theories and conclusions including my 29-year self-experiment with DHEA.

Yet, in seventy-odd years of life, I have dealt with or witnessed a range of illnesses and conditions. I've also written this book in consultation with a retired physician MD and sought his insights and approval. Anyone who takes action based on my findings here is operating on their own judgment and risk.

Another important point: Anyone currently under treatment for a disease should NOT substitute my DHEA approach, or discontinue treatment, without first consulting their physician. I would never try to advance a "quack treatment" for illness, one that supplants or interferes with established, real medicine.

A good deal of medical treatment later in life involves mitigating the ill effects of aging. Therefore, it goes without saying that mature people could save substantial medical costs if they avoid these ills. Fortunately, medical practice involves a sacred oath to act for the benefit of the patient, and to do no harm. I would not anticipate a harsh reaction or retaliation to my crusade to rescue humanity from the terrors of old age and death.

A question arises which is typically the first assumption or challenge I face when I state my theory: "If your method is so simple, safe and easy, why has no one thought of it before?

Haven't all the wise researchers already scouted this and ruled it out? Who are you to fly in the face of centuries of science research? A mere nobody, trying to revolutionize medicine?"

My answer is, there has to be a discoverer. It often takes, not a specialist building on known science but a generalist, a renaissance rogue thinker, to reverse conventional thought and see the new paradigm. The inventor of handwashing, as necessary for medical treatment and surgery in the mid-19th century, was universally rebuked, ridiculed, and denounced as a crackpot. He was resented by those who could not contemplate changing the old views, until handwashing became the usual and required practice.

As an interdisciplinary Conservation student at Berkeley, I was taught to step back, look for hidden patterns, and discern new relationships in an ecosystem or a landscape. All of that may have paid off in a few small ways, including my revolutionary help alleviating symptoms of the common cold and my immortality regimen.

Back then, "thinking outside the box" hadn't even been invented.

Another factor: I was lucky to receive a hint at a crucial time from a bestseller, hearing Dr. William Regelson speculating over the radio about the possibilities of DHEA. As Lewis Mumford quoted, "The way to rise highest is to stand on the shoulders of giants."

Still, there remains the question: Why is DHEA an "orphan drug," ignored by medicine? The usual reason for saying this is that a drug can't be patented and therefore cannot lead to monopolistic price-fixing by some "Big Pharma" drug maker. This is true of D; it can't, as a substance already natural to the human body, be patented. It is available in the US without prescription from many pharmaceutical sources. It's also not an "anabolic steroid" with a narrowly targeted market such as muscle building or athletic performance. Strictly speaking, it's not even a drug, just a supplement.

But the main factor with DHEA as a medical substance is the dosage. It isn't usual or practical for an MD to prescribe a drug in gradually increasing doses. But in my regimen, our "need" or tolerance for D builds steadily with aging after our prime. This isn't a self-generating habituation, like addiction to opiates, but rather it results from an increasing natural deficiency. It's not "megadosing" a pill like Vitamin C to fight colds, since my regimen starts with a tiny dose for optimal effect, with no rush or giddiness craved or chased. We're now told that, because of excess drug and vitamin intake unused by the body, our urine is the richest ever, polluting waterways and mutating fish; but this wastefulness shouldn't be the effect of careful D self-administration.

Prescriptions are typically for a fixed amount over a definite time, subject to renewal in a year or two. A nurse or MD may occasionally administer a drug such as a painkiller PRN, or As Needed. To allow a drug to be increased at will, open-ended, would be practically inviting a wasteful, dangerous overdose. Fortunately, from research, DHEA does not seem prone to overdose. (At this point, one note of caution: DHEA is a lipid fat, and it's possible for lipids to form one type of kidney stone. So, a long-term excessive dosage of DHEA, more than the body needs or consumes, might speed up the formation of painful stones. Thus, the importance of a gradual and internally validated increase over the years.)

So, an MD has difficulty recommending more DHEA based on subjective feelings, without a blood test. And worse, a test result of "Normal" is often based on age, but without designating for what ages, on the results readout. In my fifties, when I finally asked what age, I was given a printout showing that my blood D level was Normal for a 19-year-old! A desirable outcome, but no help if a catastrophic drop in DHEA level is reported as Normal for a seventy-year-old. Which in fact it is.

It seems likely that, based on further research, guidelines can be made available showing typical declines and dosages for advancing ages at one-year or five-year intervals. But individuals may vary, especially over a thirty-year term of decline, so such a chart would be at best a rule of thumb. And if you wait for blood testing to show a deficiency, theoretically you're suffering age damage until your dose is adjusted. That's why I hope that my subjective sensitivity to a morning shortage can work for others too, as a daily check to maintain or

advance their dose.

PILLS, ETC.

In the interest of full disclosure, here is a list of my three doctor's prescriptions, plus any meds and supplements I've taken in the last dozen years, since age 65 (I now take only ten or so of these):

DHEA, self-prescribed, increased over the years from approximately 12 to 600 mg. daily

Avodart or Dutasteride 0.5 mg. daily: Prescription for BPH (benign prostate hypertrophy)

Super Beta Prostate, beta sitosterol supplement, 2 or lately 3 pills daily for BPH (Note: I tried to quit each of these two remedies, but I need both to control urinary function and comfort.)

Alpha lipoic acid: temporary supplement advised by a podiatrist to help with peripheral neuropathy

L-methyl folate: a form of folic acid, same as above, helped to relieve foot twinges

Afrin nasal decongestant mist, oxymetazoline HCL: nightly only, clears sinuses to prevent snoring

Glucosamine supplement for joint healing (I don't add chondroitin due to a mild shellfish allergy)

Aleve/naproxen: painkiller for knee pain and tenderness; bad choice for a torn meniscus (recommended by a doctor and taken for a year; meanwhile, my joint damage grew worse)

Turmeric: herbal supplement for joint healing

Boswellia Serrata (frankincense), ditto

Bromelain (pineapple extract) ditto

Piperine: (black pepper extract) ditto, often in combo pills

UDC-II: undenatured collagen from chicken cartilage, daily to halt osteoarthritis immune attack

Eggshell membrane pills: glycosaminoglycan proteins daily to hydrate and cushion cartilage

Resveratrol: mitochondrial cell energy booster derived from red wine

NAD: Nicotinamide Adenosine Dinucleotide energy booster (not nicotine, declines with age)

Vitamin A, alternate days to avoid overdose: supplement for night blindness while driving

Vitamin D: supplement for limited solar exposure in northern latitude (doctor recommended)

Vitamin E for healing, NOT. I quit this on hearing it may block prostate meds. No change seen

Vitamin K cream: salve to repair deep skin layers on back of hands from long-term sun damage

Orange pulp and juice with citrus bioflavonoids: food to prevent and alleviate hand bruising sooner

Aspirin: occasional anti-inflammatory painkiller for bee sting, headache, etc.

Collagen: I try to supplement this from Jell-O, though I often neglect to prepare it

Retinol oil: I've applied this to wrinkled or sun-damaged skin. Some wrinkles went away for good

CBD: non-narcotic ointment for muscle and joint strain and nerve pinching, frequently used on pain

Levothyroxine 75 mcg daily: <u>Prescription</u> replacing normal thyroid hormone loss due to aging

Anastrozole 0.5 mg daily <u>Prescription</u> to balance body's testosterone conversion to estrogen: DHEA gives me high-normal or excess testosterone, per my blood tests. But my body converts excess T to estrogen. If E is high, I feel lethargic; but with too much testosterone, I'm irritable. So, I balance them with a tiny dose of Anastrozole, 1/2 mg. daily. It limits my body's conversion of T to E but sustains the amiable disposition I've always had. Suggested by an endocrinologist & prescribed by my regular GP.)

NOTE: Some of the above items, often regarded as palliatives, may have enhanced or more permanent benefits for me due to my DHEA supplementation and healing.

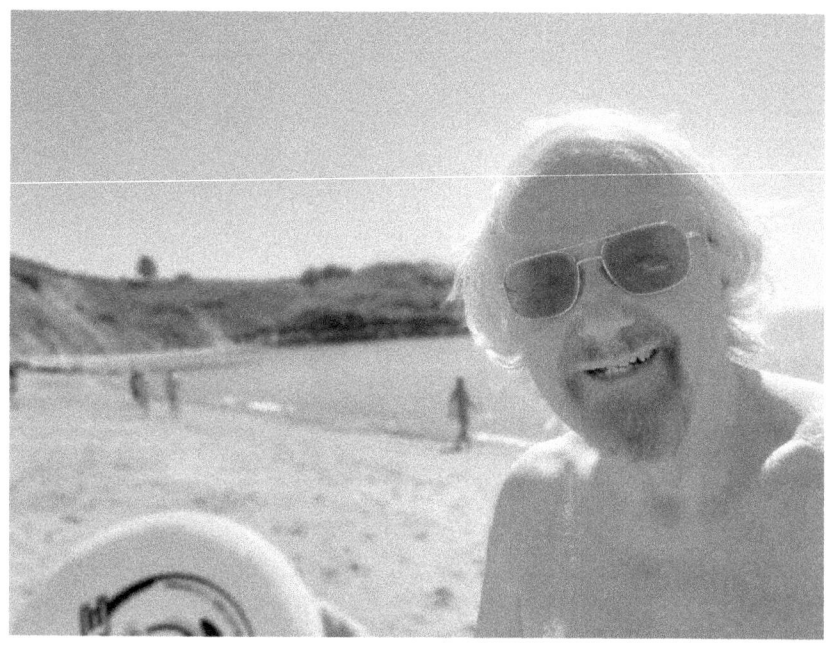

CHAPTER 10

MY STORY

EATING DISORDER

Born in 1948 in Chicago, Illinois, in boyhood I was puny, 40 pounds by age 8. I lacked a healthy appetite, so much so that my divorced father took me away from my mother, who couldn't make me eat. Mom wasn't much of a cook, and I remember hiding Brussels sprouts and cut-up bites of Swiss steak in our telephone cabinet rather than chew them. The foods that I best remember (besides penny candies and popsicles) were sardines and Norwegian Fiske Boller (codfish balls from a can), an occasional feast of boiled shrimp (my dad joked that I was a cannibal, a shrimp eating shrimp) or rolling white "balloon bread" into dough balls, or dipping crackers in milk and eating them soggy.

School lunches in Chicago were tiny red hot dogs cooked tough and chewy on a dry bun. Food at home was overcooked, tasteless, and irregular. My big, rare treat was running downstairs with a dollar for "hot tamales" from the cart of the old Mexican street vendor.

At age 8, on a two-week summer trip out West, Dad drove me all the way to the Pacific Ocean and kept me. He gained legal custody in California, and there we found real tamales, spaghetti, chili burgers, hotcakes and other foods that I would eat, even vegetables (or else, he decreed, sit and stare at them until they dry up and blow away!) My scrawny size became a legal issue, and Mom didn't effectively contest Dad's custody claim. I did return to her for one summer, and there at age 10 I ate most meals with her tenant family downstairs, who served me soups, good seed bread and Lithuanian cheese. I didn't mind eating, and their old lodger Adolph taught me to chew each bite thirty times.

Back in California, I remained skinny but became active. I learned to ride a bike, played outdoor games other than snowball fights, and took Scout hikes. I was treated for allergies with weekly shots—possibly to validate my father's custody claim. But I haven't suffered from seasonal allergies.

VISION, HEARING, ALLERGY AND SINUS

Finally at age 11, after chronic strep throat that kept me out of school for weeks at a time, I had a tonsillectomy during a year that Dad and I spent in El Paso, Texas. There I improved, wearing nothing but a pair of cutoff jeans while playing outdoors and roaming the desert most seasons.

My long strep absences from school, with lots of reading, made me studious, a teacher's pet. My vision was poor, nearsighted with an astigmatism, until Dad got me eyeglasses. Myopia is genetic and progressive due to the shape of the eye sockets. It's still with me, but my eyesight stopped deteriorating twelve years ago. My hearing loss inherited from Mom, which began about age 60, stopped by 70; my hearing aid and eyeglass prescriptions haven't changed in ten years.

My allergies were never severe, with no seasonal hay fever. The main allergy was to "house dust," really the dust-mite remains prevalent in bedding, both in Chicago and Cali. Whether or not the allergy shots made a difference, I remained a mouth-breather all my life until my fifties, when I began clearing my sinuses before bed with Afrin or Sinex nose spray to relieve snoring. This was further improved in my sixties with the use of mite-proof mattress and pillow covers. My continued allergy to the tiny arthropods also makes me slightly sensitive to shellfish. And one of my daughters, an identical twin, has a severe allergy to shrimp, even the cooking fumes, that can lead to anaphylactic shock and medical emergency. (Her twin, strangely, seems to lack the allergy but has suffered mild asthma.)

I also spent many adult years with an undiagnosed sinus infection, finally cleared out by the latest antibiotic. My lungs are usually very clear with the help of the nose spray, and by breathing steam vapor, coughing and spitting in the shower. Occasionally, since I never smoke anything, doctors will tap endlessly at remote parts of my back while sounding me out with a stethoscope, thrilled by the echoes. From boyhood I heeded Mad Magazine, whose satirical ads often targeted smoking.

I haven't developed any new allergies with age, except possibly to bee stings. Last year I went out to get my mail in stocking feet. There on my front walk, I was savagely stung by a dead bee, already dry and shriveled in dead leaves. The side of my foot hurt, itched, and swelled slightly; but the stinger came off with the sock, and I recovered in a day. Then two days later, extreme swelling and sensitivity returned. It had to be my immune system kicking in, releasing the new antibodies. I didn't see a doctor but got relief in a day or so with aspirin and cold packs on my foot. The violent reaction shows how active my immunity remains at age 76... a good thing really, in this era of new infectious diseases, so long as I stay clear of a "cytokine storm" immune reaction, now treatable with immunosuppressants.

PHYSICAL DEVELOPMENT

As a boy I didn't do well in sports—apart from a try at football, breaking my collarbone—until I took up Frisbee and pool diving late in high school. Afterward I enjoyed back-country hiking and camping, swimming and diving in cold High Sierra lakes.

Later in my thirties, I qualified as a Wham-O World Class Frisbee Master, with one appearance in the Rose Bowl Tournament. Also, in 1974, my new wife and I bicycled for nine months throughout Europe; we later backpacked across the Grand Canyon and the High Sierras. From high school we were together for fifty years, with three children. But never trying DHEA she died of ovarian cancer in 2014.

Long before D, I was fortunate to have no serious injuries or illnesses. I broke my collarbone diving for a football, and my nose in a school fight. And much later I broke my ankle rescuing a kitten, all bones adequately reset. I suffered mumps,

chickenpox, and plenty of colds and flu, until I learned to fight

them off by gargling salt water and immediately sucking on

zinc lozenges to head off the virus.

DENTITION

My teeth had numerous cavities, with metal fillings that still hold up. That was exquisitely painful, but NOT because of the drilling and filling. As a young college stop-out, I'd been couch-surfing at my fiancé's pad, neglecting to brush my teeth for a month or so. (When I first had 'em cleaned in Berkeley, it was so excruciating that I actually feared the lovely young dental hygienist was a sadistic Nazi torturess. And her attitude toward me, as I squirmed and tried to escape, was suitably vengeful.)

My neglect of dental care was partly rebellion against my dad. He wanted me to become an orthodontist, but my ambitions were mental, not dental. When I finally got dental coverage, I had several cavities in my molars, so the young DDS put in wide fillings to cover and protect any surface that might possibly decay and spare me any more fillings. As a result, my teeth were extremely, keenly sensitive to heat and cold. And, fortunately or not, my new job was in a hospital, living and dining on the grounds. Their cafeteria had requirements that the steam-table food must be served HOT, and the milk and beverages COLD. To a twenty-year-old with a big, urgent appetite, it was torture. For years, wolfing down delicious, nutritious meals. I learned to pucker my lips around my teeth to reduce the shock, and to drink through a straw, never with ice, till finally the misery declined with blessed age.

I've had no more fillings and only one that broke. I had one cracked tooth replaced at age 72 by an artificial molar, rather than going through a cap, root canal, eventual extraction and bridge. Apparently, I've had no bone loss; my new dentist, unable to extract the broken tooth, wore himself out over at least forty minutes drilling the root out of my jaw. I suffered no significant pain then or now. Recently, it may be possible to head off tooth sensitivity and cracking with "densifier" enamel-building toothpaste.

AGING

Since starting DHEA in 1996, I've overcome many common issues of aging: Hearing, and vision loss corrected with eyeglasses or contacts; Prostate trouble, whose cause isn't yet fully understood, controlled with pills; Kidney stones, mainly oxalate, not lipid, passed or hypersonically fractured; Hair graying, easily addressed with color secrets made Just For Men; Joint damage always a risk, but worse due to extreme showing-off; Shingles, often triggered by stress, now vaccinated; Sleep disruption—mainly due to being a writer able to work anytime in bed, like today at 5 AM; Hair loss that still seems to threaten... but then, it always seemed to. As early as high school, seeing my widow's peak, a friend proclaimed, "Leonard has a receding hairline." Insulted, I responded, "It's not receding, it's staying right where it always was." And there my hairline remains. I do notice some hair loss, especially in dry weather, but there's still enough to sustain my sparse surfer-wave. It may help that, for prostate ills, I take Avodart (dutasteride) by prescription, a drug that is sometimes abused as a hair restorer.

Luckily, as a retired, leisured male, I've been able to overcome the above challenges with medical help and coverage or reduce them to a mere nuisance level. First, with eyeglasses or contact lenses and ever-cheaper hearing aids. And now, teeth and gums can be protected by new toothpastes, including enamel-builders. I'm lucky in that if I use plaque-fighting toothpaste, I never require cleanings. I no longer even need to floss. Dental hygienists complain that my teeth are too clean.

KNEE JOINTS

Joint damage can become severe if wear and tear exceeds the cartilage's ability to heal, such as from extreme jobs like athlete or firefighter, or from sports that may be addictive, like jogging or snowboarding. They say the cartilage in large joints, like knees, is slow to heal due to a lack of circulation; but it can indeed heal from nutrients in the synovial fluid. In youth, with my wife, our months of steep pedaling under load in Europe did no discernible damage. But later in life, I challenged my knees excessively to show off, by jumping from walls and fences while retrieving frisbees, pedaling too hard on hills, etc. One Halloween, while lurking on my porch roof to light the jack-o-lanterns, I spied a bunch of teenage trick-or-treaters running around in my front yard. Unable to resist, I leaped down into a clear spot in their midst, a foolish and potentially

crippling risk to my back, if not my knees.

Luckily it had rained heavily, and the lawn was very soft.

And I—in addition to my vampire cape—was wearing pixie

boots with three-inch heels. Those heels sank deep into the soil,

absorbing much of the shock. But as the adolescents scattered,

I also heard a crack in my back.

Years later, a young local recalled the Halloween frolic in

my yard, when a caped figure appeared from nowhere and they

all ran for their lives. I was able to assure him I was alive, not

undead. But occasionally I did have mid-back twinges; and

later when a chiropractor x-rayed my spine, I saw that one of

my vertebrae is missing an ear-tab. So, I got away with it,

once; no telling what that spinal disk would do if I tried such a

foolhardy trick again. Immortality in a wheelchair would be

less fun.

As part of getting younger, I later aggressively tried to recover the full-squat ability that I'd lost even before starting DHEA. To flex my knees, I did duck-walking, with the water supporting part of my weight, in my shallow backyard pool. But I also did squat-jumps across the narrow ditch in my genius self-designed plastic pool, which may have aggravated the cartilage wear. And the hula hoops, too, probably weren't best for overused, thinning knee cartilage. Not to mention stand-up sex.

Before long, I had a torn meniscus in my left knee with occasional, burning, bone-on-bone contact or extreme weight-bearing pain. It likely became a "bucket-handle" tear, where a strip of cartilage can double-over for enhanced agony. Some mornings I'd wake up feeling fine, but experience an intense, burning pain the first instant I flexed my left knee before synovial fluid was drawn in to lubricate the bone-on-bone contact. For my earlier inflamed, tender touch pain on the proximal (inner) side of that knee, a GP had recommended a regular over-the counter pain pill, naproxen (Aleve). But such an NSAID (Nonsteroidal Anti-Inflammatory Drug) pain reliever probably wasn't the best idea, because it killed the pain of all my foolish activities, instead of letting pain slow me down. Chronic pain can be nature's way of telling you, don't blow it, let it heal. And limit the use of painkillers.

Fortunately, my minor injuries were seldom severe enough to involve the addictive risk of opiate pain drugs. My only involvement with opiates was to reset a broken nose, and for kidney stone pain. Those brief encounters with morphine and hydrocodone were enough to scare me off with their power.

It took me two stem cell shots (costly, and not covered by insurance) endless joint supplements, and a year or two without any running or bicycling to heal my osteoarthritis, torn meniscus, and later a jammed right knee from a fall. I had to do careful research and take an active role in choosing therapies to heal my knees, now almost fully restored. In so doing, I rejected a "scrape" (curettage) and artificial knee that was foretold.

Yet I believe that this full healing might not have been possible in a normally aging person, without my DHEA regimen. I was told by a surgical nurse that I would have artificial knees in two to five years. That was nine years ago. Now I run, bicycle (fast but sanely) and catch Frisbees again. But to this day, I still get occasional warning knee twinges around both knees, reminders to go easy.

A freak accident to the right knee set back and restricted my athletics for a year—probably to the benefit of my left knee, which needed time to recover from its torn meniscus. To avoid kicking my wife's laptop by its dangling cord onto the bathroom floor, I took a fall on my left arm and right knee. The arm recovered, but the knee didn't, disabling me for a whole weekend, and forcing me to walk with an antique crooked cane my brother-in-law Lou had crafted for me. Months of cramps, halts and twinges ensued, along with a third stem cell shot to soothe that right knee. Forget running, climbing ladders, bicycling or crouching in a squat ever again!

Only now, years later, am I back on bikes, chasing Frisbees and boomerangs, on and off the roof, and duck-walking in the pool (buoying up part of my weight to get closer to a full squat.) Would this recovery, while living a full life (with many foreign trips, and later during Covid restrictions) have been possible without DHEA? And without evident aging?

From a medical research standpoint, in evaluating a drug or treatment, it's important to learn the patient's (or the research subject's) family and personal medical history, plus their lifestyle and habits.

These can introduce extraneous factors or "confounding variables" that skew the results.

For instance, in my case, the fact that up through middle age, I lived a moderate lifestyle—with an ample and varied diet, no obesity, no smoking, very little alcohol, no coffee, cola or caffeine (limiting even chocolate due to my allergy test), no narcotics and no long-term medications—those facts should contribute to my longevity. My one indulgence would be challenged nowadays as a sweet tooth, since I never tried to avoid candies, cakes and ice cream, but remained active, and didn't need to limit calories. Through late middle age, I even avoided soft drinks with modified corn syrup in favor of natural fruit juices. That was when I had children in the house and was concerned about their sugar intake.

So, the question might be, have all of my healthful efforts warded off aging and kept me youthful, INSTEAD of my steady DHEA supplementation? Am I a sterling exception? Or just genetically lucky? Do these "confounding variables" negate the findings of my self-experiment?

My answer is No. Experience shows that the most extensive health program of the most dedicated fresh-air fiend cannot significantly extend the human lifespan. Sure, we may avoid or recover from diseases of aging, fight off, or even reverse weakness, shrinkage, and senility briefly, but the best habits and the most massive medical interventions cannot vanquish death—until now.

Only by replacing and sustaining a single molecule, DHEA, can we overcome nature's lethal plan. Loss of D is the simple, elegant kill-switch that starves every organism to death. I would surmise that, with DHEA supplementation, any number of "bad habits" might NOT prevent D from sustaining and prolonging a reprobate's lifespan—although I dread to think of anyone harming his or her body with bad habits, suffering irreparable damage, and then condemned to live forever with the ills and regrets of their self-destructive behavior. I wouldn't wish that on anyone.

CONCLUSION

In Conclusion, it seems fitting to list those common problems and infirmities of aging I DON'T suffer:

COVID: Wife and I fought it off with salt gargle, zinc lozenges, expectorant fumes, etc., and later tested negative. See Final Bonus Chapter 12.

Diabetes: none, and no family history, including Adult Onset Type 2, now often called "Diabesity." I do have a sweet tooth for candies, pastries and drinks. Luck, or DHEA? NOTE that Diabetes 2 onset (Adult Diabetes) typically occurs around age 45. It might be alleviated or blocked entirely by replacing DHEA, which helps to regulate insulin production.

Obesity: never. For years at 5'11", with daily weigh-ins and skipping meals, I've kept to 170 lbs.

Heart disease: none; my pulse is regular, about 75 beats per minute at rest.

Blood pressure: normal, under 130 systolic when tested.

Cholesterol: high normal, with a high ratio of "good" HDL cholesterol to "bad" LDL.

Sarcopenia: no apparent loss of muscle mass or strength.

Skin: no sags, wrinkles, crepe or veins, except sun-damaged wrists (Note: my left hand is slower to heal from bruising than my right. USA drivers get more cancers on the left / sun-exposed side of faces, arms, etc.) The bruises are called senile or solar purpura.

Vitamin K cream, and consuming citrus pulp bioflavonoids, seem to relieve this for me. The damage, cumulative over decades, seems repairable when treated while taking DHEA.

Bruising is rare, paler, disappears faster, and a severe bruise lasting years finally cleared up!

I carry sunblock in my cars to protect the backs of my hands and wear garden gloves.

Veins: no phlebitis or edema. (Veins visible only on hands due to sun-damaged fair skin).

Bone loss: no sign of osteoporosis fragility during falls, somersaults, bone drilling, etc.

Height: my driver's license height at age 20 of 6'1" is now constant at 5'11" for many years.

Skeleton: my lifelong "dowager's stoop" is much improved with physical therapy this year.

Spine: I've overcome issues with my lower, middle and cervical spine including scoliosis. (Lower back twinges with medical marijuana; middle with PT; scoliosis with chiropractic).

Neck: improved rotation and motility after PT last year, from a pre-DHEA neck injury, 1992.

Incontinence, Irregularity, Night Enuresis: None, with prostate remedies. Latest PSA 2.58.

Sleep: as a writer my hours are irregular but never wasted; no long-term deficits except jetlag.

Alcoholism: occasional limited drinking, if followed by water intake, yields no hangovers.

Sexual function: normal, recently steady over 8 years with my 25–33-year-old ex-wife/lover. Frequency, alone or mated, is at least twice a week.

Viagra: Seldom used because it causes me mild gastric reflux/heartburn.

Vertigo: Only rarely, due to other causes (BPPV, meds, jetlag) now quickly overcome.

Healing: Blood clotting, immune reaction, and skin knitting all unimpaired.

Inflammation: With daily turmeric and antioxidants, I believe there's none present in my body.

Apnea: When I clear my sinuses and sleep on either side, no complaints of snoring.

Teeth, hair, vision, hearing: corrected, with no losses in last 12 years. 1 cracked molar, replaced.

Peripheral neuropathy: minor, due to a drug, treated by a podiatrist within the last ten years.

Mental acuity: greater than ever, as evidenced by this book and the novel I'm also writing.

Memory: comprehensive but not always instantaneous. Trivia is "not deleted but delayed".

Mood: more stable and positive than ever, except regarding current global threats and crises.

Social skills: still learning and improving, I hope. I try to entertain.

Arthritis/rheumatism: none; my past ten years have been a gradual victory over osteoarthritis.

Graying: corrected monthly or so, but there remains some blond color in my body hairs.

Cancer: none yet, with regular checkups against Dad's prostate and Mom's colon cancers.

Pain: no chronic pain, rare positional neck pain from a spine injury while lifting furniture.

Brain: no headaches except sinus congestion due to dehydration or hangover, alleviated by drinking water.

Energy: normal, with occasional TV naps or mild couch-lock in the late evening.

Cataracts: "Who gets cataracts? Only people with birthdays," they say. But I've no sign at 77.

Night blindness: I've heard that the surest way to estimate someone's age is to shine a light into their and observe how quickly the pupils contract. But with a Vitamin A pill every other day, I have no difficulty driving at night with oncoming lights, except during a torrential rain.

I attribute the absence of all the above ills to healthy living, medical monitoring, AND DHEA.

So, as Conan's Valeria said, "Do you want to live forever?" As our parents say, "Never get old!"
UPDATE: This sounds too good to be believed. In 2023 I suffered what I call my "achy-breaky neck" syndrome from

excessive computer use, querying 250 literary agents from my bed. I had quit my joint pills, so it caused arthritis in the tiny facet joints of my neck: chronic pain, corrected by January 2024 with physical therapy and supplements. It still took months of good posture and exercise to heal. But the PT ALSO corrected my old C7 neck injury, treated in 1992, AND has straightened my lifelong "dowager's stoop" hunchback. I no longer sleep on a special pillow, high on the right and low on the left, to wake up without numb hands. I've regained full neck rotation since the "incurable" disk/cartilage/pinched nerve injury to my neck. I stand straight now, getting younger! Thank you, DHEA!!!

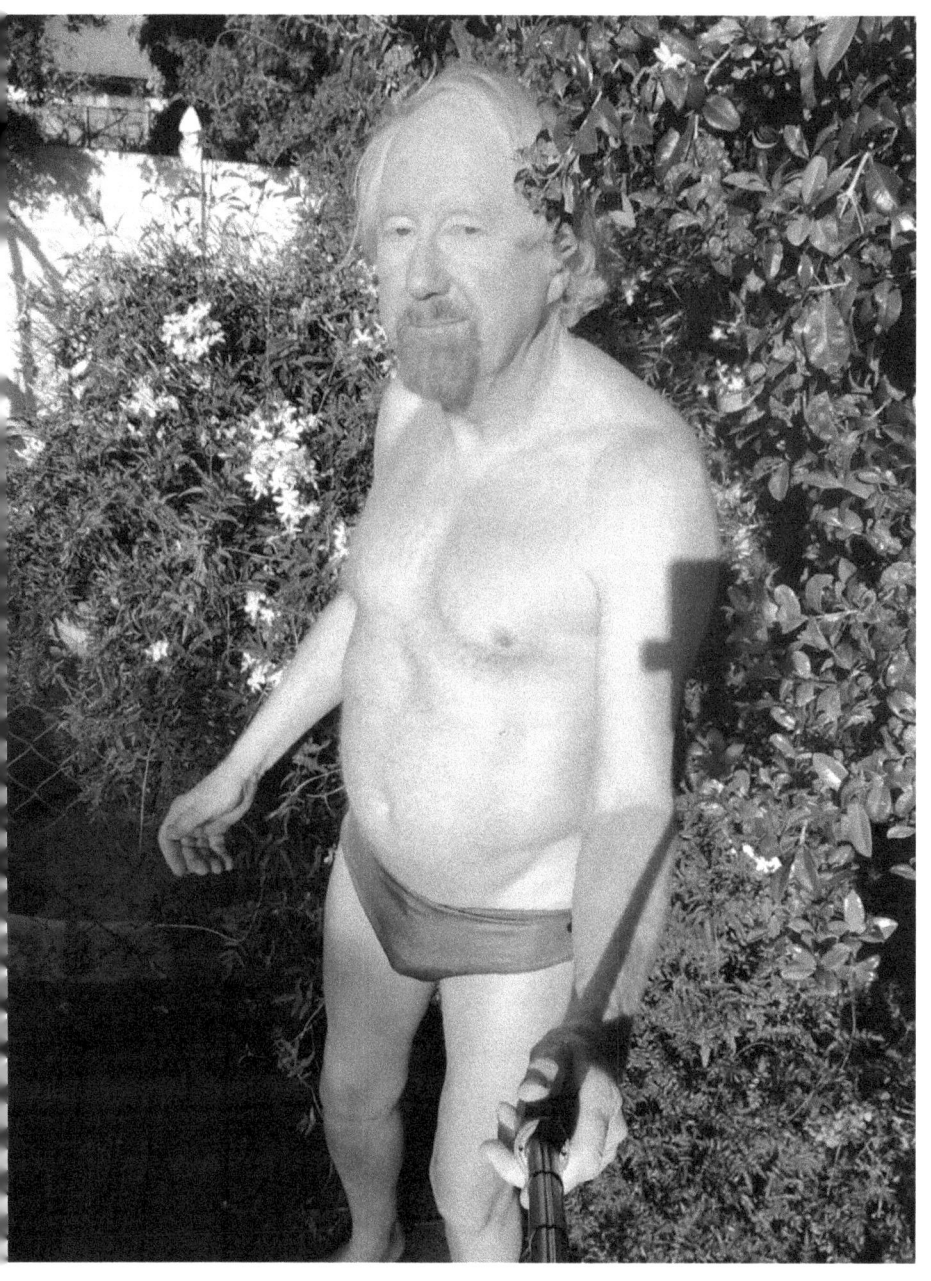

CHAPTER 11

Q&A: In Conversation with Leonard Carpenter

Question by a reader: So, Leo, you're saying at 45, I'm the right age to supplement DHEA?

Answer: Maybe, with your doctor's okay. I can't be that precise, but your feelings should tell you.

Q: Well, of course I'm getting older. But I've got a lot on my mind lately.

A: As a family man, you mean? I get it. That's when the kids leave home... or don't! And our parents grow old and infirm or even die. We worry about losing them; meanwhile we learn about the ills and terrors of aging. Some of us go from parenting our kids to parenting our parents, or both!

Q: I never had to think about aging. Now it's all that older people talk about, and all over the TV ads and dramas. What happened?

A: That's my generation's fault, the Baby Boomers. We suck up all the air. My old friends are all aging out, but we have so many anti-aging products, programs and exercises to extend our lives and use up the last of our money. We were in denial before, and didn't even plan to live past 30.

Q: Physically, I don't feel that old. Why should I even worry about it?

A: Yes, exactly! Well into middle age, I was in the my prime of my life. Stronger than ever, smarter but facing new challenges. I learned computers and ended up working for kids half my age; I had to stay young to be employable. Then at 48, I began commuting weekly to LA and couldn't juggle sleep and driving so well. I felt old.

Q: That's when you started DHEA?

A: Yes. By luck, I heard about it on the radio. It was mentioned in a bestseller back then in 1996, and the author was riffing on its potential. From my motel, I walked across the street to Longs Drug Store and bought it.

Q: And so, it helped your endurance, your stamina?

A: Evidently. After a morning pill I felt normal, youthful all day No buzz; I didn't drink coffee then.

Q: So, just one pill a day worked?

A: Yes, but even then, I figured on gradually increasing the dose. Dr. Regelson on the radio had explained, DHEA naturally declines in your body with age. So that was my plan, to steadily replace it. But in fact, I had to decrease my dosage right away.

Q: Because of side effects?

A: Yes, sort of, too much effect. After that first week feeling young and energetic, I knew DHEA was working. And if I skipped my dose, I felt a definite lag by noon, the familiar old age; I had to take a pill later to feel normal again, right away. But then one morning after a week of whole pills, I felt jittery, nervous, too hormonal. Oh, and I got a pimple on my face! I didn't want to be THAT young, so I began cutting my pills in half.

Q: And that worked? Half a pill a day?

A: Yes, for a year or more, I felt normal, energetic. Driving, working, writing my book, homemaking on weekends. Only much later did I begin feeling draggy and old after my morning dose.

Q: So, you went back to a full pill?

A: Yes, for a day. But that was still too much! I felt jumpy again, wired to the ceiling. So, I cut the half-pills in half and took three-fourths of a pill for a while. From 25 mg. down to 12.5, then up to about 18.75 milligrams. Not weighing it, just splitting the pills evenly. Now it's easier to use liquid DHEA, with a graduated eyedropper for exact amounts. But half and quarter pills were ballpark for me, with good results.

Q: Then back up to 25 milligrams?

A: Yes, after a year or less. Whenever I felt a lag, I upped my dose to feel normal, and no jitters. The increases became larger and more frequent, but I hardly noticed from year to year. By age 60 I was ordering 50 mg. capsules by mail, then 100's. The price didn't go up much for the extended youth and health benefits. And the exact sensitivity of those first feelings and needs, so steady and reliable, just validated to me that my hormone replacement theory was working.

Q: Your natural DHEA was declining faster?

A: I had to think so. Looking back now, I see it really dropped off in my sixties. Then I was going up in my dosage by 50 or even 100 mg. at a time to stay youthful. But into my early seventies, I no longer felt any lags. For years now, I've been steady at 600 mg. per day. I tried increasing to 650 last year, but felt no boost, and no real deficiency.

Q: So, it's been, like, perfect health all along?

A: God, no! (Laughs) As a DHEA pioneer, I was always challenging myself to prove how young I was. I vaulted fences and jumped off sheds, recovering Frisbees. I pedaled extra hard instead of shifting bike gears. I would throw disks and boomerangs, then run to catch them myself, stopping on a dime, violent exercise. I also had a lot of past knee strains, bicycling thousands of kilometers in Europe, and then to and from work for various jobs. By age 68, I had torn cartilage in one knee, then a worse injury to the other, both putting me onto a crutch for days at a time.

Q: So, you've had knee replacements, implants?

A: No, I canceled surgery and instead shelled out thousands for stem cell shots. I took it easy for a few years, stayed off the bike and let the dog chase the Frisbees. I also treated myself, first with painkillers, NSAIDs – which was a mistake – but also joint supplements, Glucosamine, Turmeric, Boswellia, etc.

Q: So you were, like, a shut-in?

A: Actually, no. I traveled to Ireland, Spain, and Cuba a dozen times in six years, hauling my luggage and trekking cities, hills and jungles. But always taking a dozen pills each morning. I think the DHEA made me more responsive to the stem cells and supplements. So, I healed faster, like a young person.

Q: You traveled alone?

A: Or with girlfriends. In Cuba, I met my 25-year-old Guantanamera and brought her home to marry.

Q: No problem with marital relations?

A: Not with a hot Cubana, no way! But I do try to avoid the Viagra, it gives me heartburn.

Q: Any children?

A: No, I had a vasectomy after my third child in 1989.

Q: With your previous wife? Did you two separate?

A: No, Cheryl died of ovarian cancer in 2014. She never did believe in my youth pill or try it.

Q: You didn't keep trying to persuade her?

A: No, it was an experiment. It took me years to feel sure that it was working. And I didn't know much about female hormones, except the hell of menopause. Too bad, DHEA might've headed off her cancer.

Q: I've heard it has anti-cancer properties. But is DHEA safe for women?

A: Yes, under a doctor's supervision, but NOT for women who are pregnant or lactating or for children. DHEA is often prescribed for female hormone replacement. In Europe, it's called Prasterone. and can be given as a vaginal salve or suppository to ease menopause symptoms.

Q: But not so much here?

A: Well, now it is. But it boosts estrogen, that some women are afraid may cause breast cancer. I've read that it's a misinterpretation of a Woman's Health study in 2002, that it was really progesterone supplementation that raised the cancer risk. By the time Cheryl's ovarian was diagnosed, it was too late. Chemotherapy kept her vital for a year. Then I retired to help care for her during her last year.

Q: So, it sounds like you then had a whole second life.

A: Yea, I'd hardly even kissed a girl other than Cheryl. So, after grieving, I relived the sexual revolution that we'd had just between ourselves, as young hippie lovers.

Q: Now you're saying any man or woman can have a new life, with or without a faithful partner?

A: Yes. One thing about DHEA, it restores all the sex hormones, so men and women don't lose interest. At least that's what it did for me. I wanted to try it out with an older woman, say, fifty-ish. But they all were know-it-all skeptics and preferred to let aging take its toll. And my Cubana's too young to need it.

Q: Have you had many believers try to follow you?

A: No. I've only proclaimed it since 2020, first with a series of Medium blogs. I had no replies except from an Italian guru guy, and one lady planning to stay young with Essential Oils from Biblical times. My TikToks as Leo the Immortal went viral, but only with brief kudos, and then Elon Musk trying to sell me Bitcoin.

Q: Why don't people believe you?

A: Well, as a writer I don't have a wide social circle. My brainy friends tend to be hard-bitten skeptics, atheistic and opinionated. They say, who the hell are you, to turn all medicine and human belief upside down? You're not a doctor or professor, not even a lab technician, so why should I believe you? You call yourself a Renaissance Rogue, the Most Interesting Man in the World, like the Dos Equis guy!

Q: You don't have any medical training?

A: Just two years as an orderly on a Geriatric Ward, which taught me a lot about old age. No miracles there, just the very basics.

Q: Why no study of medicine?

A: Medicine is a tight discipline. They train you to think a certain way. A doctor prescribes a fixed dose of meds for the duration of an illness or forever. The idea of slowly increasing your dose is unsafe, just asking for addiction or an overdose. And too, doctors can't expect patients to monitor their own state of health, except for occasional meds that are prescribed PRN, as needed, and usually given by a nurse. Nurses like the ones I used to work with are sometimes the most in touch with everyday reality. To deal with the essential, hormonal nature of life and death, I needed to think outside the box, beyond usual professional medical limits. Still, I need to regularly check with medics for new developments and keep from violating medical principles or taking undue risks. Luckily, my pill was simple and safe, a natural substance taken orally, that's most abundant in the youngest, healthiest human bodies.

Q: So, DHEA isn't an anabolic steroid? You invite no heart issues or 'roid rage?

A: No, it's a precursor, a basic ingredient that your body can transform into whatever hormone the organs or tissues need at the moment. If your hormone balance is healthy to begin with, your system will tend to preserve that balance. Ask my friends, I haven't changed much in fifty years. Hormone injections, like testosterone, will definitely change your body's balance, not always for the best.

Q: Are you addicted to DHEA?

A: Alas, no. It would be easy for me to quit – like, if I went on a trip and lost my pills. But I'd start to feel old, weak and spiritless. I think my body would soon be taking on aging damage that could become permanent. That's one experiment I never tried, quitting for more than two days! I didn't like the result.

Q: So, you have to be diligent about taking your pills?

A: Yes, that's the challenge. Most people, if they're feeling crummy, will take another cup of coffee, another smoke or energy drink, or a puff of weed. That palliates the sense of aging, covers it up, but it doesn't arrest aging. And all those quick fixes have risky side effects. I now can enjoy coffee, alcohol in moderation, even weed, if I want to watch Aquaman and forget it again! But I'm in touch with the baseline of my hormonal well-being, first thing each morning when the body's hormones, if any, are released, and I supplement them with my pill or powder. If the DHEA habit is working, you recognize a steady, gradual need. No frequent changes.

Q: Then a doctor can't tell you how much to take?

A: I now have annual blood tests for male hormone levels and show them to my GP. One test, when I was about sixty, said I had the DHEA level of a 19-year-old. But since then, the results are age specific and I'm well over the limits. I hope that someday, after long-term studies, the DHEA decline of different individuals, male and female, can be charted and some guidelines established. My feeling was my mood and stamina were just fine until I faced extra stress and exertion at age 48. My own feeling has been the best judge. If anyone else chose to follow in my footsteps, I'd hope to offer inspiration and reminders, and even supply the product through my website.

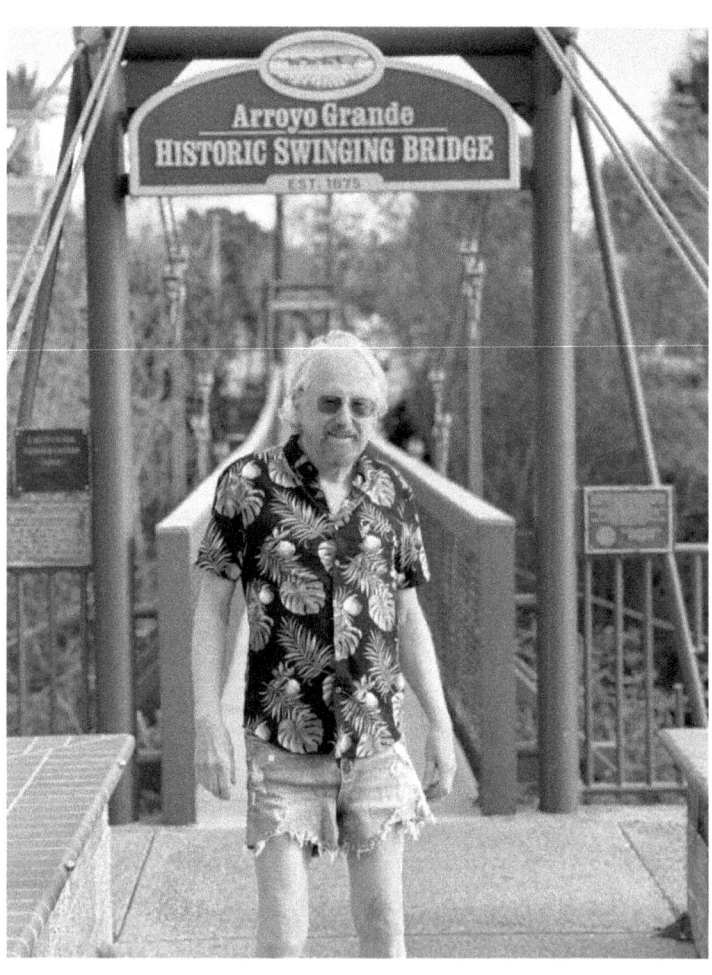

CHAPTER 12

Leo's Genius Ideas for a preventative approach to the common cold (and other respiratory ills)!

(What is genius? It's seeing what may have been overlooked by others. LC)

What's this, another cheap, easy, do-it-myself panacea for one of humanity's worst problems? This original remedy of mine, mentioned in passing earlier, deserves a full explanation. Like my DHEA treatment for death itself, it results from a simple insight, just a careful dosing of known, safe ingredients.

Again, this remedy is from my own experience. It has worked so far for me, no guarantees. Here's how I found it, by luck and genius.

Once during a flu epidemic, I asked my doctor, "Bob, tell me: you see a dozen sick patients a day, and you don't even wear a mask. How do you keep from getting the flu yourself?"

His reply was, "Simple, I just gargle with salt water between patient visits. That gets rid of any virus exposure."

Easy for a doctor, I thought, who pops in and out of your life in his own office. But other docs had suggested this, and I was intrigued. "How does that work? Does salt kill the virus?"

"No,' he said, "it draws them out, by reverse osmosis. Your throat is a semi-permeable membrane, so you just spit out the viruses and they're gone."

It took me days to figure out what he meant. I recalled a chemistry experiment in high school. Our teacher, Mr. Mills (we called him General Mills) showed us a glass tank divided in the middle by a thin membrane, maybe parchment paper secured by tape. When he added salt to one side of the tank and stirred, the paper bulged away from the salty side. The brine was expanding, drawing in more water to dissolve the salt, by creating "osmotic pressure." The paper was permeable to water but not to salt, so the other side remained freshwater, although shrinking. (The volume of the few spoonfuls of salt wasn't enough to make it bulge so much, especially since the salt was dissolved in the water, in solution.)

Viruses, I learned, aren't even living things in their dormant state. They're just complex crystalline molecules that can flow along with water and pass through the semi-permeable mucous membrane of the throat. They only behave like living predators once they're injected into live tissues. There they swiftly replicate, cannibalizing the cells.

Still, the osmotic pressure of the salty water can draw the virus particles back out of our throat tissue with other fluids, preventing their replication. Doctors say the water needn't be too salty, just a level teaspoon of salt to a cup of water. When first mixing the two, using warm tap water can speed up dissolving the salt, but stirring also works. If the salt taste is too unpleasant, I immediately rinse it off of my taste buds. But I let the solution linger awhile in my throat by extended gargling.

So, when I feel any throat irritation, that first step is gargling and spitting, at least twice to cover all of the infected tissues switching from left to right. I try to exhale nasally and lean forward, letting the salt water penetrate into, and flow out of, my nose, if possible, through both nostrils into the sink.

After gargling with salt, I feel immediate throat relief. But that's just half the battle. Now comes Step Two, the double-whammy. It's zinc, a metallic element which blocks the cell receptors that viruses seek to "dock" onto.

It seems clear to me; every airborne cold or flu virus goes for the throat. The mucous membranes of our throat, upper respiratory tract, and sinuses: that's our "Achilles heel." It's the

place to detect, fight, and stop the attackers dead. It's advisable

to keep zinc throat lozenges close at hand.

I once had a dear old friend Carlisle, who took zinc

gluconate pills for good health. But instead of swallowing

them, he sucked on them. I tried the pills (clearly labeled and

non-prescription) once or twice, but found they had a foul taste.

My old pal always had very bad breath. Clearly his pills were

meant for internal use, likely to remedy some zinc deficiency

real or imagined, not as lozenges.

But as I later read, zinc in the throat can help to resist throat

inflections. Unlike the soothing cough drops of my youth,

effective against hoarseness or dry throat, or just to ease

coughing, zinc lozenges can keep viruses from attaching and

reproducing. Nowadays, brands like Cold-Eze come in pleasant

flavors with no aftertaste. The ads say, in language approved by the FDA, those lozenges can shorten a cold. I say, immediately after salt gargle, they can lick a cold or flu well before it overcomes the initial immune response and gets a foothold in your tissues or bloodstream.

To be effective, the drop should be in the throat a few minutes. For repeated bouts to head off a virus, I often suck up half of a lozenge, then rewrap it for the next round. I always carry salt and zinc lozenges with me when traveling; I'm tired of hunting though dark hotel kitchens by night in quest of salt.

I try to act logically while fighting a cold: it helps to stay hydrated, especially to flush out mucus, but drinking or eating should be done BEFORE gargling so as not to wash away the benefits of salt and zinc. And by staying with the fight, I can usually feel relief within an hour or so.

I find it's important to act promptly, at the first hint of throat distress. Alas, if I don't end up getting sick, I can never be absolutely certain that it worked, except maybe in the unique case of Covid. But in the last dozen years, only one cold has snuck through to plague me.

On my TikTok stream I include a vivid re-enactment of our Covid attack, a battle fought along with my 30-year-old wife who suffered identical, simultaneous symptoms. Our fight was desperate, because it required four or five rounds of gargling, between our onset of throat and bronchial distress at eight PM on a Saturday night, and 2 AM next morning when we beat the virus. We'd obviously both been exposed at the same time, possibly on our New Year's Day trip to Disneyland.

Our symptoms and reactions were unique but identical: the sudden sick feeling, fevers, and thick, stringy mucus clogging our bronchioles, markedly different from the usual scratchy throat irritation. Had we chosen to sit and wait in a clinic or emergency room at that late hour, we likely would have swiftly fallen ill. But luckily, I had my trusted, proven protocol to meet the challenge.

Between bouts of gargling and zinc-ing, we had to cough and spit aggressively to clear our lungs. As I had rarely done in the past to fight off or recover from lung congestion, we lay upside-down off the end of the bed with a box of tissues, letting gravity help us spit out phlegm. We had no Vapo-rub as an expectorant, so I had to drive to a nearby eucalyptus grove and cut off fronds to boil. Then, bending over the kettle with towels draped over our heads, we took turns breathing the soothing, liquefying vapor. Then more spitting, gargling, and lozenges until we felt healthy.

By the wee hours our breathing was clear, with no other symptoms. We went to sleep and awoke feeling fresh. The Emergent Care we went to said we were too healthy to waste then-rare Covid tests on. But we had no relapses, and my blood later tested free of Covid antibodies. Since then, I've been diligent in keeping up with my vaccinations. Covid can be especially tough on elder victims.

Our therapy worked because my genius combo punch defeated the strategy of the viruses. That is, to replicate swiftly, much faster than our immune systems can awaken and dispatch antibodies to neutralize them. By stalling the onslaught one or more times, and thus slowing virus multiplication, we could allow our own immune systems to take full effect. That was equally possible for my 30-year-old wife AND for me, with my 71-year-old immune system maintained at full strength and readiness by my longtime replacement dosing of DHEA.

This simple cold prevention technique, my invention, is easy to try and can yield quick, impressive results—as a precaution to try while waiting for a medical appointment! I hope it inspires readers to give my DHEA anti-aging method a fair hearing.

Never get old!

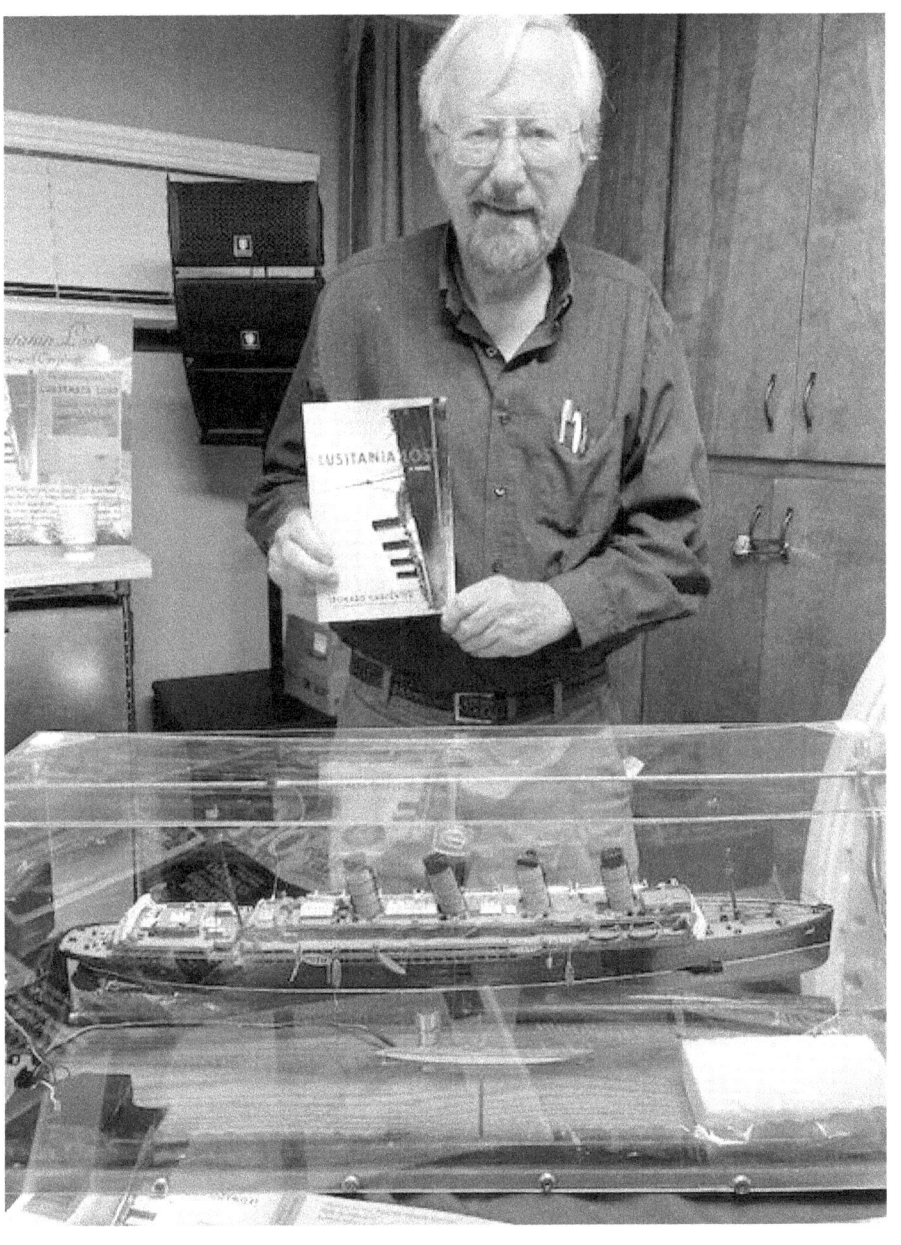

BIBLIOGRAPHY

alpha by title

A Review of Age-Related Dehydroepiandrosterone Decline and Its Association with Well-Known Geriatric Syndromes: Is Treatment Beneficial? Rejuvenation Research, 2013 Aug; 16(4) pp. 285-294 (A study relating partly to cancer treatment)

DHEA The Youth and Health Hormone

C. Norman Shealy, M.D., Ph.D.

Keats Publishing. Los Angeles CA1999 (A pamphlet book describing DHEA's benefits and decline)

Estrogen Matters

Avrum Bluming, M.D. and Carol Tavris, Ph.D.

Little, Brown, Spark, New York NY 2021 (An excellent

authoritative account of estrogen's benefits)

Lifespan: Why We Age, and Why We Don't Have To

David A. Sinclair, Ph.D.

Atria Books, Sydney AU 2019 (Attributes aging largely to

DNA and telomere damage.)

The Aging Clock

Walter Pierpaoli, William Regelson and Nicola Fabris

Annals of the New York Academy, 1994 (a very technical but

inconclusive collection of research)

The Case For DHEA (free Q&A pamphlet listing research on

the safety and benefits of DHEA)

Altea Health, Olympia WA 2019

https://www.fitnessquest.com/wp-content/uploads/2020/11/The-Case-for-DHEA.pdf

The DHEA Breakthrough

Stephen Cherniske, M.Sc.

Ballantine Books, New York NY 1998 (This original research doesn't promise immortality)

The Metabolic Makeover: It's All About Energy!

Stephen Cherniske, M. Sc and Natalie Kather, MD

Altea Media LLC, Olympia WA, 2014

(Remarks by Dr. Kather: The benefits of DHEA, this important human repair signal, still remain a secret to many. Despite over 10,000 studies about DHEA readily available to the public, it remains an enigma to many of my medical doctor colleagues. I have been supplementing my DHEA to get into the health zone for women over two decades, as measured by blood testing. My husband Stephen has been supplementing for 38 years to keep his DHEA level in the health zone for men.)

The Metabolic Plan

Stephen Cherniske, M.Sc.

Ballantine Books, New York NY 2004 (More strategies including DHEA for extended life & health)

The Superhormone Promise

William Regelson, M.D. and Carol Colman

Simon & Schuster, New York, NY 1996 (Introduces Melatonin and DHEA)

END NOTES

* regarding broad claims. Other content is based on the author's personal insights.

Chapter 2 – Regelson, p. 43

Chapter 2 – Rejuvenation, p. 2

Chapter 2 – Regelson, 43 et seq.

Chapter 2 – Rejuvenation, p. 3

Chapter 2 – Shealy, p. 1

Chapter 3 – Shealy, p. 44

Chapter 6 – Bluming, p. 196

Chapter 6 – Shealy, p. 27

ACKNOWLEDGMENTS

My personal physician, Dr. Robert Okerblom who never discouraged my longevity experiment.

To Teri Bayus, my Book Manager, who shows me the way.

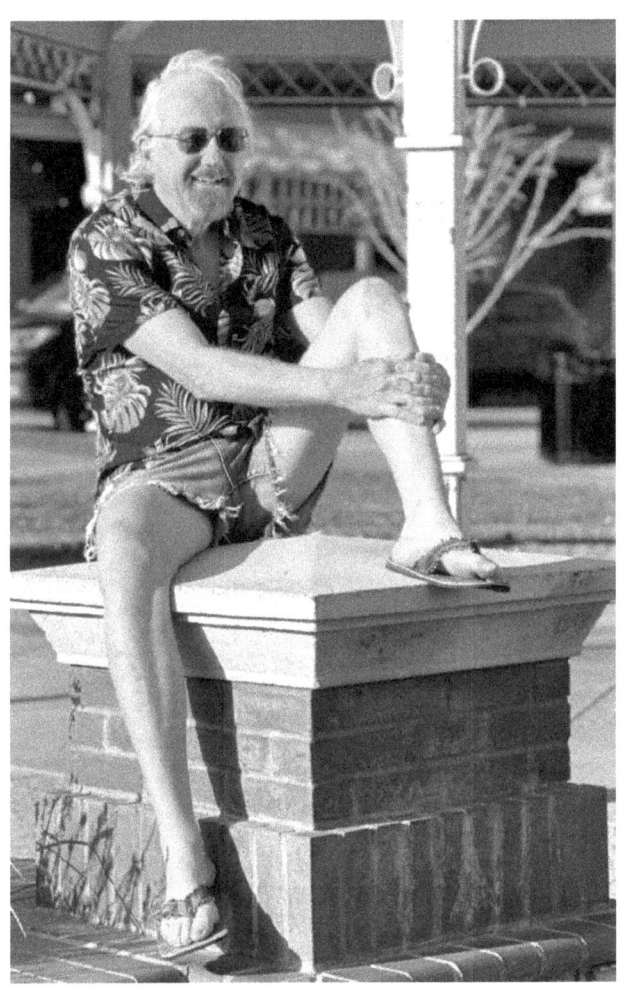

CONTACT

Website: www.dhealthy.net

Email: leonard@best1.net

Contact- Website: www.leonardcarpenter.com

TikTok: leosimmortaltales

Published By:

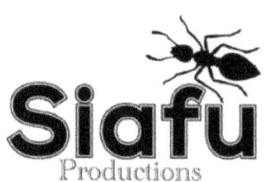

ALSO BY THE AUTHOR:

Lusitania Lost: A Historical Novel
https://a.co/d/82XjCCb
A World War I spy thriller from an author who puts "electrifying action into everything he writes" (Jonathan Maberry, New York Times–bestselling author).

Alma Brady is on the run from a New York mob boss. Desperate to escape Big Jim Hogan and his murderous gang, she joins a group of nurses bound for the Great War in Europe. Their ship is the Lusitania, the most celebrated luxury liner of 1915, with a passenger list of Broadway and Continental celebrities—who do not realize they are headed for certain doom.

This epic sea romance portrays the events surrounding the Lusitania's final voyage, from the White House to the mean streets of New York, to the palaces and battlefields of Europe. With President Woodrow Wilson, King George the Fifth, Kaiser Wilhelm and the young Winston Churchill as characters, the unfolding drama explores all the circumstances that brought America into the Great War, including some mysteries that will never be solved.

Biohacker
https://a.co/d/9FO8AEK
Fans of Outbreak, Contagion and Inferno will thrill to the enigmas of this futurist medical mystery!

Biohacker, set in 2035, is an intimate medical thriller about a designer plague. The anonymous computer and gene hacker, a physician/stalker obsessed with reducing Earth's population, announces his intent in highly personal emails to journalists Will and Eva Warner. They soon realize that the plague's creator, the self-styled Biohacker, must be one of the medical team they've been helping to fight the Blackpox epidemic. But which one, and to what sinister purpose? Meanwhile romance, obsession, climate peril, computer intellect and the world's largest aircraft Skyport play their fatal roles.

Conan the Renegade
https://a.co/d/hYsu9fs
A Hyborian sequel honoring Robert E. Howard's legendary character
Conan, becoming leader of Hundolph's mercenary company, revolts against the ruthless betrayals of Prince Ivor, fights strange new sorceries, and soon runs afoul of an ancient curse.

Conan The Raider
https://a.co/d/1JFZIec
Venturing south to the warring lands of Shem and Stygia, Conan forms a plan to rob the Tomb of Kings, at the unimaginable risk of awakening their Undead Armies.

Conan the Warlord
https://a.co/d/5yrF1vu
Conan, plucked from a dungeon to serve as the double of Baron Einharson's dissolute son Favian, soon has ideas of his own on how to lead the kingdom against the rebel armies of the serpent god Sethissa.

Conan the Hero
https://a.co/d/7bgBMVs

Conan as a mercenary captain finds himself violently and romantically involved in a jungle drug war. From afar in the Turanian capital, Emperor Yildiz observes and gives reason to say, "Don't be a hero!"

Conan the Great
https://a.co/d/91og9PP
Conan, newly crowned King of Aquilonia, faces untold rivals out to seize his realm: the armies of Koth, Ophir, and Nemedia joined under the generalship of the ruthless young schemer Armiro; Kthantos, an all but forgotten god; the violent seductress Amlunia; and Delvyn, the fool.

Conan the Outcast
https://a.co/d/1fPWGSD
The ancient hierarchs of the desert city of Qjara did not want the young man called Conan of Cimmeria inside their walls with his strange, northland ways. He did not even worship the One True Goddess. Yet some would ensnare him in the city's intrigues: the beautiful Princess Afriandra, with powers she does not fully understand herself, and Zaius, foremost swordsman of the Temple Warriors. Their paths are like nothing Conan has seen before, following labyrinthine trails he cannot imagine, thrusting him toward banishment or death. And in the dying city of Sark, the soulless High Priest Khumanos wields the legendary Sword of Onothimantos and schemes for the return of ancient gods. Qjara does not want Conan, but only one man can prevent the sacrifice of the city to Votantha, the Tree of Mouths. Only one, Conan the Outcast.

Conan the Savage
https://a.co/d/9xTBcd2
After a gambling dispute erupts in violence and death, Conan of Cimmeria is condemned to the hellish mine pits of Brythunia which no man has ever escaped, nor survived. But Conan breaks free and disappears into the wilderness, far from **civilization** and into the eager arms of Songa, a forest maiden. Still the demon-goddess Ninga has seized control of Brythunia, and her insatiable appetite for human sacrifice threatens to devour the world. Only one man can strike at the very heart of Ninga's religion of blood. A man who carries death in his eyes, and vengeance.

Conan the Gladiator
https://a.co/d/2Tt4NHK
Lured by a beautiful acrobat, Conan becomes the strongman of a traveling troupe, only to end up as a gladiator when his company is forced to fight in the Circus Imperium, a wonder of Conan's Hyborian world.

Conan of the Red Brotherhood
https://a.co/d/7aFy88v
While the decadent Emperor Yildiz and his corrupt allies plot the destruction of the barbarian now known as Amra the Lion, Conan carves out a pirate empire with the strength of his cutlass and dagger.

Conan, Scourge of the Bloody Coast
https://a.co/d/b9vVnBv
Conan, the pirate king of the Vilayet Sea, faces dangers on every side as the lure of ancient pirate treasure draws him into

conflict with the evil arch-wizard Crotalus, and into an apocalyptic battle.

Conan, Lord of the Black River

https://a.co/d/2caoo0X

Conan the Cimmerian must venture into the nightmare realm south of the River Styx to retrieve the Silver Lotus, a powerful remedy that can undo the dreaded Plague of Dreams which holds the city of Queen Rufia under the spell of the undead witch Zeriti.

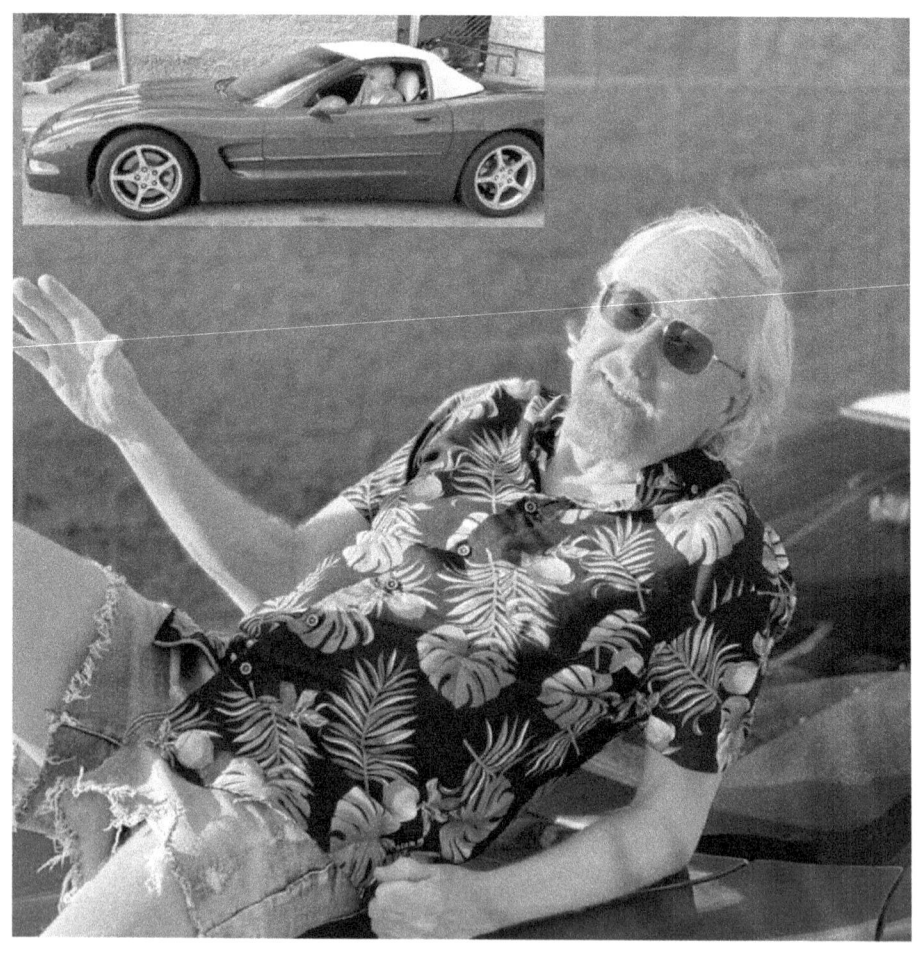